SCIENTIFIC AMERICAN

EVERYTHING YOU NEED FOR

WINNING SCIENCE FAIR PROJECTS

Grades 5-7

by Bob Friedhoffer

Illustrated by **Ernie Colon**

A Byron Preiss Book

To Ace Greenberg

As good a friend as he is a magician

ACKNOWLEDGMENTS

Annette, who lets me try my experiments at home with few kvetches. Charles Curtis, whose upbeat calls of cheery encouragement were an oasis in the desert of writer's block. Howard Zimmerman, whose advice has been invaluable in making this a better book than I could have done on my own. Nikki, who does chemistry projects every day. Madeleine, who will do some science experiments one day. Joe Kincheloe, who introduced me to Friere and Critical Pedagogy. Phil Anderson, who has been an incredible help in finding my topic. Bob Elliott, who "steals (magic tricks) only from the best." Bill Kelly, who is the guardian at the gate. Martin Gardner, who has been my muse for many years.

SCIENTIFIC AMERICAN
WINNING SCIENCE FAIR EXPERIMENTS
Grades 5–7

Copyright © 2004 by Byron Preiss Visual Publications, Inc.
In cooperation with Scientific American

Edited by Kate Nunn
Associate Editor: Charles Curtis
Cover design by Andy Davies
Interior design by Gilda Hannah
Interior illustrations by Ernie Colon

iBooks are published by iBooks, an imprint of J. Boylston & Company, Publishers.
www.ibooksinc.com

CONTENTS

BOB FRIEDHOFFER teaches teachers how to teach science in the classroom. He is also a touring, practicing stage magician, and many of his illusions represent basic science principles. Friedhoffer is a member of the National Science Teachers Association, the American Association of Physics Teachers, the New York Academy of Science, the Academy of Magical Arts, the American Federation of TV and Radio Artists, and the Screen Actors Guild, among others.

Friedhoffer's books on science and magic include: *Yet More Magic Tricks, Science Facts* (2001); *Old Magic with Today's Science* (2001); *Physics Lab in the Sporting Goods Store* (2001); *Physics Lab in the Playground* (2001); *Physics Lab in the Supermarket* (1999); *Physics Lab in the Home* (1997); *Magic and Perception* (1996); *Toying Around with Science* (1995); "The Scientific Magic Series" (1992, six titles): *Matter and Energy, Forces, Motion and Energy, Heat, Sound, Electricity and Magnetism, and Light; Magic Tricks, Science Facts* (1990); *How to Haunt a House for Halloween* (1988).

RESOURCES FOR SCIENCE FAIR EXPERIMENTS

Supplies. All of the materials required for the experiments in this book can be found at home or in "houseware supplies" stores and "hardware" stores.

Information and further ideas. It is recommended that readers visit one or more of the following World Wide Web sites for more information on the science involved in this book's experiments, as well as for ideas for other experiments in the same areas of science. If you do not have a computer with an Internet hookup at home, try your school or local library.

http://www.ipl.org/div/kidspace/projectguide/
http://www.sciserv.org/isef/
http://energyquest.ca.gov/projects/index.html
http://www.ars.usda.gov/is/kids/fair/ideasframe.htm
http://kids.gov/k_science.htm
http://canadaonline.about.com/cs/sciencefairideas/
http://www.physics.uwo.ca/sfair/sflinks.htm
http://www.cdli.ca/sciencefairs/
http://www.scifair.org
http://homeworkspot.com/sciencefair/
http://school.discovery.com/sciencefaircentral/scifairstudio/ideas.html
http://www.all-science-fair-projects.com/category0.html

A pie chart is used when measuring percentages: it splits your data into different sections like slices of a pie. The bigger the slice of the chart, the larger the percentage of your total data.

PLANT NUTRITION AND GROWTH

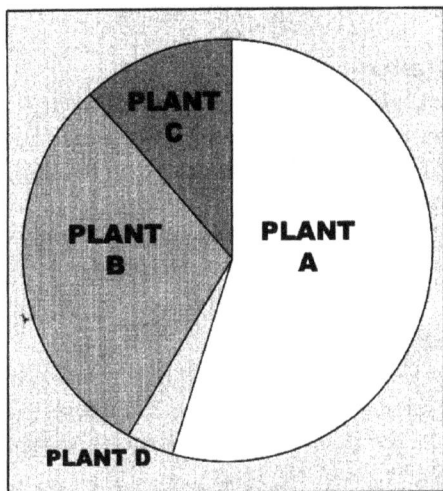

Not only should you write down all of the numerical information you get from your experiments, but you should also place all of your thoughts and observations about the project in the notebook, such as:

• What area do I want to discover something about or examine?
• What is the exact question about that area?
• Did I get my parent's permission?
• What do I think the conclusion of the experiment will show?
• Make a list of the necessary materials for the project.
• How you arranged everything to perform the experiment.
• What were the results of the experiment? How much, how far, how hot, how cold, etc.
• Was my hypothesis proven or disproven? (Either one is good.)

A Report for the Tabletop Display

Usually in a science fair experiment, you present your information as a report in sentence and paragraph form explaining everything you have written in your lab book. Start by presenting your hypothesis and explaining your step-by-step procedure of how you did the experiment. You should then display your data, followed by a section that explains what the data indicates about your experiment. Finally and most important, there should be a few paragraphs about your conclusions as you discuss whether your hypothesis was confirmed or disproven. When you finish your report, try to find a way to explain the experimental data and results on display panels. You would like the information to be easily read and understood by anyone examining the display. Displays are frequently presented as three-panel charts with the information applied as follows.

The upper portion of the left side panel usually supplies the problem/question under study and your hypothesis. The lower portion of the left side panel usually gives an overview of the experimental procedure.

The upper portion of the center panel usually has your name, the name of the project, your teacher's name, your grade, and your school name. The lower portion of the center panel is often used for charts, photographs, and illustrations. The right hand panel generally shows a summary of the data with the results you have observed and your conclusion. The tabletop in front of the three panels is frequently used to display the experiment itself. Try to make the experiment on display available to all who walk by so you can demonstrate what you have done. And have fun!

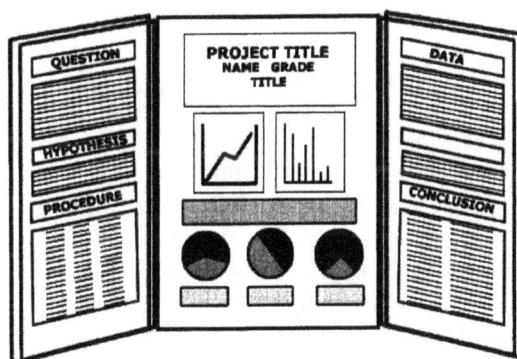

Waves, Ears and Coils

Explanation

What do music, a telephone call, a balloon burst, footsteps, and a saw cutting through wood have in common? They all have a sound associated with them. Sound is almost everywhere in our lives. Even when we try to remove sound by putting in ear plugs or wearing sound absorbing ear muffs, we can hear sounds that our body makes —the blood coursing through our veins and arteries, our own burps and our own voice if we talk out loud.

Sound waves are compression waves that travel through the air and various other substances. If you put your ear next to a metal railing and a friend taps a coin some distance away on the railing, you can hear the tapping through the railing because sound waves travel through metal.

We will be examining two kinds of waves in these experiments. The first is the transverse, the wave you see when a flag is flapping in the breeze or waves move across a body of water.

Question

Can we make our own transverse wave to see how these waves travel through air and water?

Hypothesis

By moving a tightly stretched spring back and forth we can see a transverse wave. The wave will seem to stay in one place while the wave energy moves forward.

Materials
• A helical spring toy, such as a Slinky™
• A 24" piece of string
• A microphone stand
• White masking tape

Preparation

Attach one end of the spring to the microphone stand, near the floor, with the string (a chair leg will work if you can't find a microphone stand).

Attach a small piece of masking tape firmly to one coil, near the center of the spring.

Procedure

1. While holding the loose end of the spring in your hand, stretch the spring, but allow it to stay on the floor or table. The stretched spring should be about 48" long.
2. Move your hand with the spring from side to side. The spring should start to have S-type curves moving on it. Observe the masking tape on the spring. Does the tape move forward and backward (away and toward your hand) or does it always keep the same distance?

Results

The tape and the coil attached to it should stay the same relative distance between your hand and the microphone stand. The wave energy seems to be moving straight ahead, but the waves seem to stay in almost the same place.

Conclusion

Waves move at 90 degrees to the direction that the wave energy is moving. We can see this type of wave in oceans, lakes, and other bodies of water. If a cork is floating on the surface of a puddle and we drop a rock in the middle of the puddle, the waves move away from the splash toward the rim of the puddle, but the cork barely moves forward or backward. It only bobs up and down, like the masking tape on the coil.

BACKGROUND INFORMATION

For us to recognize sound, these pressure waves must reach our primary mechanism for hearing, our ears. The pressure waves pass through our ear canal and hit the eardrum. The eardrum vibrates, causing three small bones in the middle ear, the hammer, anvil, and stirrup, to move, which causes a fluid in the cochlea to vibrate. The vibrations eventually get sent to the brain as electrical pulses. The brain then interprets this as sound.

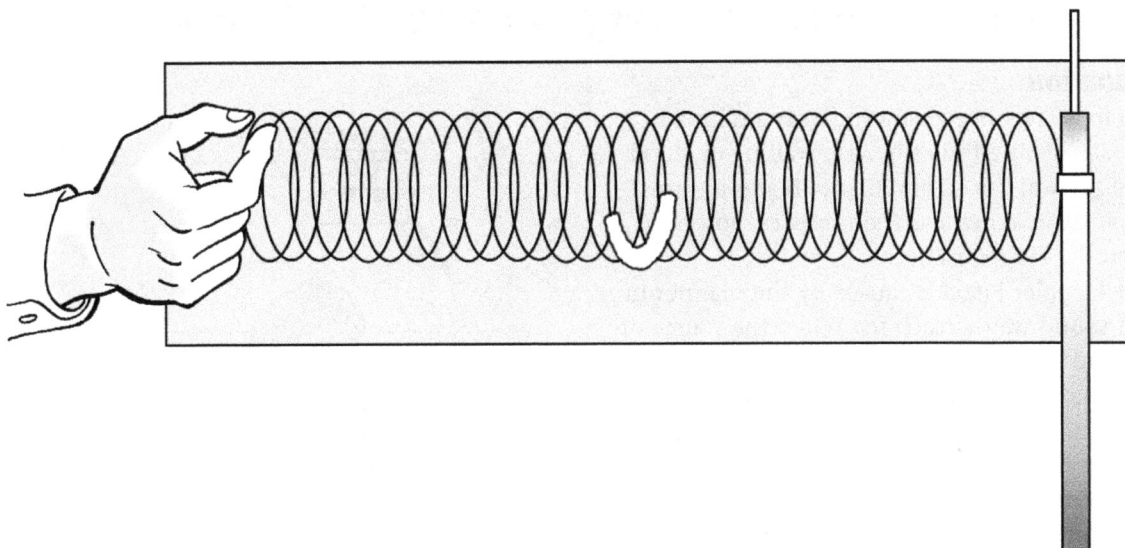

SECONDARY EXPERIMENT

The second type of wave is the kind that allows us to hear. They are known as compression or longitudinal waves. Here is an experiment that will show you how they move.

All you need is a helical spring toy, such as a Slinky™, and an assistant.

BACKGROUND INFORMATION

THE SPEED OF SOUND

If you have ever been at a ball game, you have probably seen a batter smack the ball and a moment or two may go by before you hear the sound of the ball against the bat. Sometimes when you look up in the sky, you'll see a jet plane flying overhead but the sound is coming from someplace behind the jet. The speed of light is about 186,000 miles per second. Sound moves at a measly 760 miles per hour (approximately) or 1,126 feet per second at sea level.

Procedure

Have an assistant hold one end of the spring while you hold the other. Stretch the spring so that it is 36" long. It should be flat on the table top. Grab six or seven coils at your end of the spring and squeeze them together. Release the coils. Observe the spring. What happens?

Results

The bunched-up coils open up, but the bunching-up section travels down the length of the spring.

Conclusion

This is similar to the way in which sound travels through the air. When we hear a noise, the thing that caused the noise made the air compress. Air is elastic, so it decompresses. The compression wave transfers to the air molecules around the original area of compression. This happens again and again until the sound reaches our ears.

How Sound Changes from a Moving Source

Explanation

If you have ever been standing near a railroad track as a passing train's horn is wailing or stood on the sidewalk as an ambulance blares a warning as it approaches and then recedes, you have noticed the Doppler Effect.

The Doppler Effect is caused by the manner in which sound waves reach us. When the source of the sound approaches or recedes from us, we hear a change in pitch. As the source approaches us, the pitch gets higher. As it moves away from us, it gets lower. The reason for this is a change in the sound wave's frequency.

Frequency is the measure of a sound wave's cycles per second. Different tones have different frequencies. High-pitched tones have more cycles per second than low-pitched sounds. As a sound source approaches us, the frequency increases, so we hear a higher pitched sound. As it moves away from us, the frequency decreases so we hear a lower pitched sound.

Question

Does a moving sound source sound different when the object approaches and recedes?

Hypothesis

A moving sound source's pitch varies as the source approaches and recedes.

Materials

- A strong, small, cardboard gift box
- A buzzer that works on a 9 volt battery (Radio Shack)
- A 9 volt battery
- A 9 volt battery connecter
- 12 feet of strong twine or string

Preparation

1. Assemble the battery and buzzer so that when the wires are twisted together, the buzzer sounds.
2. Place the buzzer and battery in the box. The wires, untwisted, should be outside of the box.
3. Place the cover on the box.
4. Tie the string securely around the box. (You'll be swinging the box around in a circle by the string and don't want the box to go flying off and hit someone.)

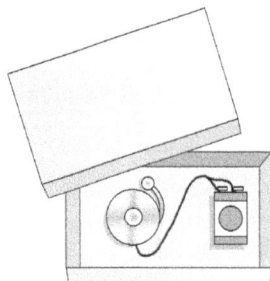

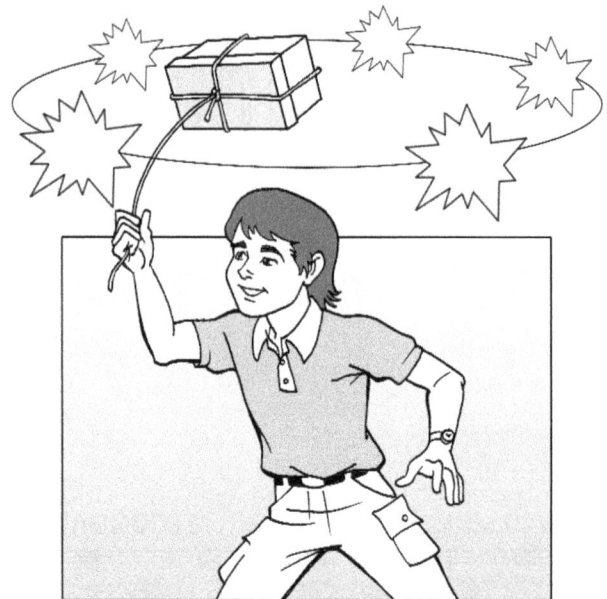

Procedure

1. Twist the wires together so that the box starts to buzz.
2. Wrap the end of the string around your hand 4 times.
3. Swing the box in a circle over your head.
4. Listen to the difference in sound as the box goes around in a circle.
5. When does the pitch get higher? When does it get lower?
6. Change the speed of the circling box. What happens?

Results

The pitch should get lower as the box starts to move away from you and should become higher when the box is coming toward you. As the speed increases, the pitch changes even more than before.

Conclusion

Due to the Doppler Effect, the pitch of a sound from a moving sound source is higher when it approaches than when it recedes. The difference between the pitches becomes greater as the speed of the object increases.

SECONDARY EXPERIMENT

The pitch of a passing sound source changes because the speed and direction of the sound source affects the way we hear the sound. The pitch is different at different speeds. Can you determine the speed of a car by the relative change of pitch as a sound source approaches? Here's an experiment you can do with an adult to find out. You'll need a driver, an automobile, 2 small cassette recorders, and 2 notepads.

Look for a secluded, relatively unused roadway, where there are no people living nearby. You will listen to and record the long blast of an automobile horn as a car drives a number of times at various speeds. You will need to find 3 easily identifiable spots along the roadway, about 50 yards apart from each other. You will be standing at the middle spot.

Note: You must stand at at a safe distance from the road when you do this experiment. Never step in front of a moving car.

Preparation

1. You will stand at the mid spot, well off the road.
2. Your adult helper should start the drive from about ¼ mile away and attain the desired speed.
3. As the car approaches the first spot, both you and your adult helper will start your tape recorders.
4. When the first spot is reached, the horn button should be activated, and stay on until the car passes the selected spot, 50 yards past you.
5. At that time, the horn should stop blowing.
6. Go through three practice runs, one at each

speed, so you will get a sense of the sound changes at each speed.

Procedure

For the experiment, there should be a least 4 runs at different speeds. The runs should be at 5 miles per hour, 10 miles per hour, 30 miles per hour, and 45 miles per hour, (or the speed limit allowed on that road). You will each record the sounds for every run on the tape recorders.

Before staring the experiment, the driver will have a note pad and write the speed he/she will be going for a particular run (Run #1, #2, #3) and keep to that speed when driving. You will not know the speed of any particular run, as the driver has arbitrarily selected a speed.

Note the speed at which you think the car is moving based on the three trial runs. Besides recording the sounds on each run, try to determine the speed of the passing car by the sound of the horn as it moves toward and away from you.

Results

You should have noticed the Doppler Effect for at least one of the upper speeds. When you listen to your tape recordings of the runs and the driver's tape recordings, you will notice a difference. The pitch of the horn as recorded in the car never changed, while there should be a noticeable change in the recordings you made when standing by the side of the road. The slower speeds had a much less noticeable Doppler shift than the faster speed.

Conclusion

The speed of a passing sound source affects the way that we hear the sound. A rapidly moving source has a frequency that increases as it approaches and decreases as it moves away. A slower moving vehicle has a much less noticeable Doppler Effect.

The difference in the way the horn sounds between the driver and the outside listener is a very basic form of relativity, as discussed by Albert Einstein. The locations of the spectators lead to different observations of the same effect.

How Does My Garden Grow?

Explanation

How do the roots and above-ground structures of plants know which way to grow? How does grass on a lawn know which way is up and that the blades of grass are supposed to grow upward? How do the roots know which way is down and that they should grow in that direction?

There are two factors involved in the growth of plants that the average person has probably never heard of: geotropism and phototropism. A tropism is a response to a stimulus.

Question

What causes the shoots of plants to grow upward?

Hypothesis

Geotropism causes shoots to grow upward. The direction of plants' growth is a response to gravity rather than sunlight.

Materials

- Beans from a seed packet normally used for growing in a vegetable garden
- 12 clean, large, new sponges
- 6 identical, large, wide mouthed jars that will snugly hold 2 sponges each
- Water
- A camera (digital will be the easiest to use for this project)

Preparation

1. Allow the beans to soak in water overnight.
2. Wet the sponges and then squeeze them to get out some of the water.

BACKGROUND INFORMATION

Geotropism (a response to the force of gravity) is the reason that most plants grow vertically. The roots go down and the shoots or body structure grow upward. For a long time, people thought that most plants grew upward in response to light. What do you think? Let's investigate to learn whether gravity or light is the cause of plants' vertical growth.

---

3. Push the sponges into the jars.
4. Push 6 to10 beans into each jar, between the glass wall and the sponges. A few of the beans should be near the mouth of each jar. The beans should be held snugly in place by the sponges.
5. Stand the jars upright and fill each one with water. Wait a few minutes until the sponges have soaked up all the water they can. Pour out the excess water.
6. Label the jars 1, 2, 3, 4, 5, 6.

Procedure

1. Keep records of where each jar is placed and its position, upright or lying down.
2. Stand one jar upright in a dark corner or closet.
3. Leave one jar on its side in the same corner or closet.
4. Stand another jar upright in a well-lit room, but out of direct sunlight.
5. Leave one jar on its side in the same well-lit room, also out of direct sunlight.
6. Stand another jar upright in a well-lit room, allowing it to receive some direct sunlight every day.
7. Allow the final jar to lie on its side in the same well-lit room, also to receive some direct sunlight every day.
8. Examine each jar every day. Make sure that none of the sponges dry out. Observe how well the seeds are sprouting in each jar. Take photos of each jar to document the day-by-day growth. Which way are the roots growing? Which way are the shoots growing?
9. Rotate the jars 180 degrees every other day. The upright jars will have a different face showing, while the jars on their sides will have their bottoms and tops switched every other day.
10. When the upright jar's sprouts are higher than the mouth of the jar, turn each jar on its side. At the same time, stand the other jars upright. Continue to observe and record

the direction of growth with both paper and pencil and photos.

Results

Most of the beans should have sprouted. The beans in the upright jars should all be growing shoots straight up and down. The roots and shoots of the beans in the other jars should have grown up and down, no matter which way the jar was turned. You should be able to tell how often the jar was turned by observing the directions of growth. When the plants were growing out of the jar, and the jars were turned, the shoots grew in an upward direction.

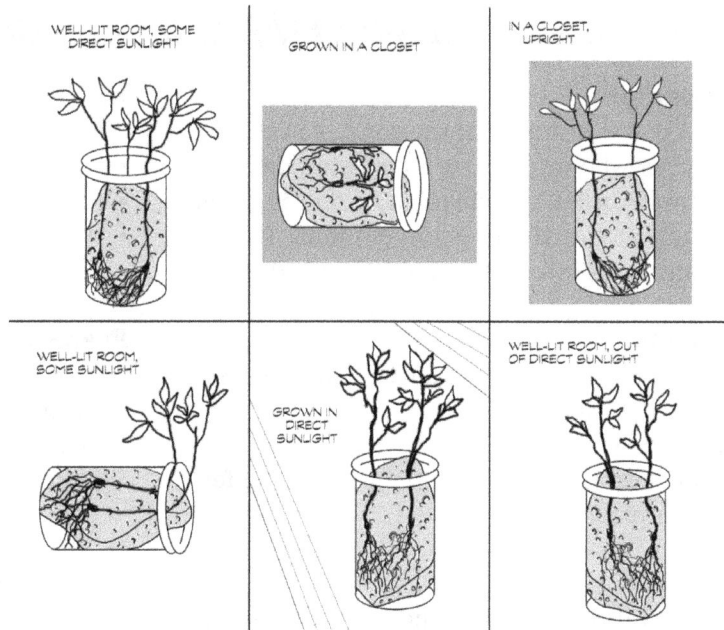

WELL-LIT ROOM, SOME DIRECT SUNLIGHT

GROWN IN A CLOSET

IN A CLOSET, UPRIGHT

WELL-LIT ROOM, SOME SUNLIGHT

GROWN IN DIRECT SUNLIGHT

WELL-LIT ROOM, OUT OF DIRECT SUNLIGHT

Conclusion

The selected plants tend to grow vertically, no matter which way their container is turned. We subjected different jars to three kinds of lighting conditions to see if light had an effect on the direction of growth patterns from just sprouting to growing as a shoot. Sunlight did not seem to play a part in the direction of growth. Gravity is probably the reason that these and most plants grow vertically.

SECONDARY EXPERIMENT

You will need three small potted seedlings of fast growing plants (from a garden store), two cardboard boxes with covers, each large enough to hold one of the plants, and a grow light.

Preparation

Have an adult help you cut a 1" hole in the side center of each box. Arrange the grow light so that it can shine directly into the hole of one box.

Procedure

1. Place one plant in each box and cover the boxes.

2. Put the third plant in a bright sunlit room.
3. Place one box near a window with direct sunlight. The box should be placed in such a way that sunlight goes directly into the hole.
4. The second box should be placed in a dark corner. The grow light should shine into the hole.
5. Observe and record the plants' direction of growth every day. Does the light seem to have an effect on the growth of any of the plants?

Results

The plant left in the sunlight is a control. Did the plant's direction of growth indicate anything? Both plants in the box should have shown a direction of growth toward the light source.

Conclusion

The direction of light can affect the direction in which a plant grows. Phototropism seems to work. This is probably why sunflowers tend follow the direction of sun across the sky, and why plants growing in dark hollows may grow crookedly.

Plant Nutrition and Growth

Explanation

Have you ever heard about someone at a state or county fair who won a prize for growing the largest watermelon or tomato? Why do you think the plants produced such enormous fruit? There are many factors that affect a plant's growth.

Question

Do fertilizers or plant foods affect plant growth?

Hypothesis

We can affect the way a plant grows by using fertilizers or plant food.

Materials

- 8 identical, small, potted, indoor plants from a gardening store. Purchase the plants at the same time from the same store. The plants should be roughly the same size, be growing in similar sized pots, and in the same general health. Plants such as coleus, African violets, or ivy are ideal for this experiment.
- 3 varieties of plant foods or fertilizers from the gardening store—not only different brands, but different formulas. (Read the lists of ingredients on the back of the boxes!) If you use organic and inorganic fertilizer, so much the better.
- Dishes to place under the plants to hold water overflow

- A camera (digital is the easiest) to help record the growth of the plants
- A ruler
- A measuring cup
- Water
- A lump of clay

Preparation

1. Find a protected place in your home where you can perform this experiment. It should be out of the way and neither too hot nor too cold. Ask your parent or guardian for permission to use the location. The temperature should be the same for all the plants (none closer than the others to a heater, air conditioner, or open window) and the plants should receive the same amount of daylight.
2. Place the plants on top of the dishes.
3. Follow the directions to care for the plants on the little tag attached to them or given to you by the people at the gardening store. The only difference in care will be the various types and amounts of fertilizers you apply.

Procedure

1. Divide the 8 plants into 4 groups.
2. Two plants will receive no fertilizer. This will be your control.
3. Three other groups will receive the three different fertilizers.
4. Use a marker pen to label each pot, indicating which fertilizer is used in it. Also, put a letter on each pot (A, B, C, etc.)
5. Follow the directions on the fertilizer container for adding the plant food.
6. Use the measuring cup to add the same amount of water to each plant every second or third day. Pour the water gently, so that you do not disturb the plant or the soil at its base.
7. On the first day, place the lump of clay next to one flowerpot. Stick the ruler into the clay so it is standing upright, 0" at the bottom 12" at the top.
8. Write the date on a small card and stand this in front of the pot.

BACKGROUND INFORMATION

There are a number of conditions that must be met for something to be considered alive in a biological sense: an item must grow, have a metabolism, exhibit motion, reproduce, and respond to stimuli. (Mules are an exception. They can't have offspring.) In addition to the above conditions, a living thing must have a cell membrane (this leaves out fire), consume both energy and matter, be composed of at least one cell, and have the ability to evolve.

This experiment examines the metabolism (the rate at which food is consumed) and the growth of plants, two of the factors that identify plants as living things.

9. Take a picture of the plant, the ruler, and the card.

10. Do the same for every plant. Continue to do this at least every third day. This will give you a visual time record of the growth of the individual plants.

11. Keep notes on how often (by date) you add fertilizer to each pot, and the days that the plants get watered. You should also keep a written record of how you think each plant, A, B, C, etc is doing. Is it healthy? Is it growing bigger than other plants? Does it look sickly?

12. After you have grown your plants for two months, collect all your data and analyze it. Which fertilizer made the plants grow the largest? Which fertilizer made the plants grow the least? Which fertilizer, if any, made the plants die? Did the control plants (the ones without fertilizer) grow better or worse than the test plants?

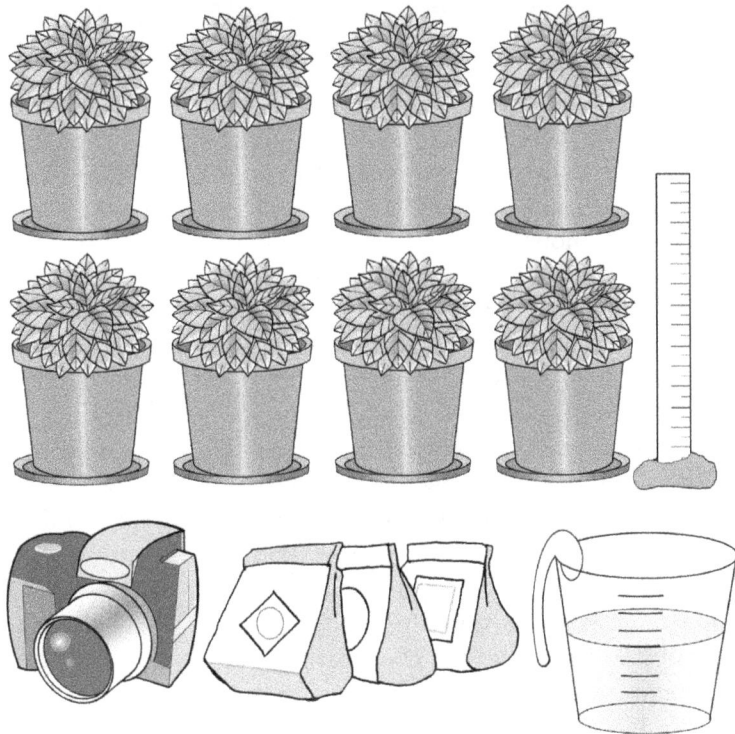

Results

Depending on the type of plant selected and the types of fertilizer used, results will vary. However, you should observe that one fertilizer is better at increasing plant growth than the other fertilizers. You should also see that the unfertilized plant did not grow as well as the fertilized plant that grew the largest.

Conclusion

Certain plant foods work best for certain types of plants, and plant food is helpful in growing large, healthy plants.

SECONDARY EXPERIMENTS

Buy additional plants of equal size and quality. Instead of experimenting with the type of plant food, you may change other factors. Feed and water every plant the same way but adjust the amount of sunlight each plant receives each day. You may do this by placing cardboard boxes or large paper bags over the plants after they have been in the sun for a measured amount of time. You could try to give one group of plants 2 hours in the sun. The others could get 3 hours, 4 hours, and no sunlight at all. Chart the results as you did in the plant food experiment.

Or you could try keeping the sunlight and plant food at the same levels, but change the amount of water each plant gets. When doing an experiment you should only change one variable at a time. If you change more than one, it is impossible to tell which change caused a change in your results.

The Collapsing Bottle

Explanation

When we ride an elevator in a very tall building, our ears pop on the way up and on the way down. The same thing happens in an airplane or even climbing a mountain. The reason is that as we rise into the atmosphere, the gas pressure exerted by the atmosphere becomes lower. The higher we go, the lower the pressure. The atmosphere ends at about three hundred miles from sea level. Babies frequently cry as airplanes descend because of the air pressure differences. They have not yet learned how to equalize the pressure by swallowing. People pass gas because the pressure inside their bodies is greater than atmospheric pressure and to equalize the pressure they must expel gas from their bodies. Heat is another factor that can affect gas pressure. As temperature lowers, so does gas pressure. Gas contracts and expands at 1/273 of its volume for every degree the temperature, measured in Celsius, falls or rises.

The colder a gas, the denser it gets, which means that it has a greater amount of atoms than a similar volume of gas at a higher temperature. The warmer a gas gets, the less dense it becomes.

Question

Does the volume and pressure of a gas decrease as the temperature lowers?

BACKGROUND INFORMATION

There are three universal measures of temperature: Celsius, Fahrenheit, and Kelvin (absolute). To calculate Celsius when we know Fahrenheit we use the formula 9/5 C + 32 = F (C= Celsius and F=Fahrenheit). To convert Celsius to Kelvin/Absolute we add 273 to the Celsius temperature. 0 degrees Celsius = 273 Kelvin. -273 Celsius = 0 Kelvin or Absolute 0.

Hypothesis

The volume and pressure of a gas decreases as the temperature lowers, whereas the volume and pressure of a gas increases as temperature rises.

Materials

- Three clean, empty, identical plastic soda bottles with screw-on caps
- An insulated bottle such as a Thermos™
- Hot tap water, the hotter the better
- A Styrofoam™ soda cooler
- Ice
- Room temperature water
- A funnel
- A waterproof garbage pail

Preparation

1. Fill the Thermos™ with hot water.
2. Fill the cooler halfway with cold water and ice.

Procedure

1. Push one bottle into the cooler and allow it to fill with ice water.
2. Place the funnel in the mouth of one of the bottles.
3. Fill the bottle with room temperature water.
4. Place the funnel in the mouth of the third bottle.
5. Carefully, so you do not burn yourself, fill this bottle halfway with hot water.
6. Allow the bottles to sit for few minutes.
7. Observe the shapes of the bottles. Are they all normal?
8. Pour all the hot water from the just-filled soda bottle into the garbage pail.
9. Hold the bottle upright and tightly screw the cap on.
10. Do the same with the two other bottles.
11. Push all of the bottles into the cooler for a few moments.

12. Remove the bottles from the cooler and examine them. Observe their shape. Are they normal, blown up or squashed?

Results

The bottle that had been filled with hot water should be squashed. The other two bottles should be relatively normal.

Conclusion

When the hot water was poured from its soda bottle, it heated the bottle and the air inside the bottle. The air expanded and some of it escaped through the mouth of the bottle. When the cap was screwed on, air could no longer enter or leave the bottle. When the bottle was placed in the ice water, the temperature of the air inside the bottle decreased. As the temperature decreased, the air inside compressed, and the volume of the air decreased. The room's air pressure was greater than the pressure inside of the bottle. The higher air pressure outside of the bottle squashed it.

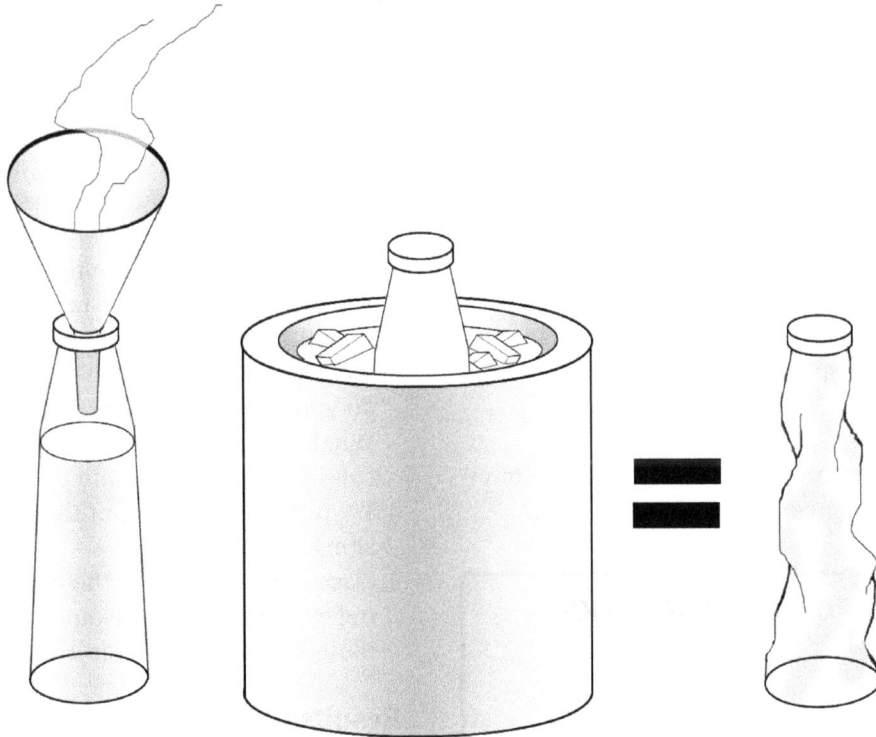

Orbiting Planets and Amusement Park Rides

Explanation

A misnamed phenomenon exists that helps us dry our clothing, perform loop-de-loops on roller coasters and also keeps the Earth from falling into the sun. The principle we commonly call centrifugal force is not actually a force. A force is a push or a pull.

Centrifugal force is a combination of two things: the inertia (an item in motion tends to stay in motion unless affected by an outside force) of a moving object and a force (centripetal force) causing the object to move in a circular manner, generally around a fixed point. This circular movement is called rotational inertia.

When a bucket of water is turned upside down, the water falls from the bucket, right? This is because of gravity. But if you swing the bucket in a vertical circle the water will stay inside. Rotational inertia forced it to the bottom of the bucket, and the centripetal force of the bottom pushed back against the water, kept the water from leaving the bucket.

When people are in a roller coaster car and the car makes a big loop that turns them upside down, why don't they fall out? The combined actions that we call centrifugal force keep the riders from getting splattered on the rails.

Question

Can we demonstrate centripetal/centrifugal force under everyday circumstances?

BACKGROUND INFORMATION

The Earth is screaming through space at 67,000 miles per hour (107,870 km per hr.) Okay, the Earth doesn't really scream. But it does move along at a pretty fast pace. If the Earth is so massive and going so fast, why doesn't it go flying off into space, leaving the sun far behind? The sun attracts the Earth, and the Earth attracts the sun because of gravity. The gravitational pull between these two bodies is the centripetal force (center-moving force) that keeps the Earth in orbit around the sun.

Hypothesis

Devices can be constructed that will not only demonstrate centripetal force but can also measure it.

Materials

- 2 identical high-rimmed paper picnic plates
- Scissors
- The cardboard tube from a roll of paper towels
- A ruler
- A flat, wooden tabletop
- A large marble or small ball

Preparation

Cut a pie-shaped wedge from one of the plates and place the plates on the tabletop.

Procedure

1. Place one end of the tube on the inside rim of the uncut paper plate. Hold the tube at a shallow angle, about 15 degrees, to the tabletop.
2. Drop the marble into the tube. When it comes out of the tube onto the plate, it should spin around the inside of the rim.
3. Put the cut plate on the tabletop. Set up the tube the same way as above, with the tube's mouth near the cutout. Drop the marble. What do you think will happen? What does happen? What happens when the marble reaches the cutout after going around the rim?
4. Try to follow the path of the marble as it goes along the table top.
5. Place the ruler next to the line of travel. Repeat the experiment. How would you describe the route of the marble after it leaves the plate?

Results

The marble followed the rim of the circular plate and moved in a circular motion until it stopped. When the marble dropped onto the cut-out plate, the sphere first moved in a circular manner as with the first plate. When it reached the cutout, it exited the plate and continued across the tabletop in a straight line.

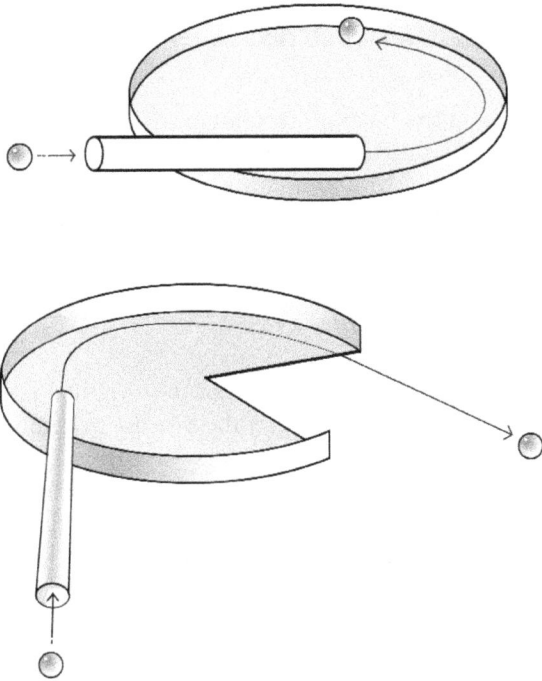

Conclusion

The rim of the plate imparted a centripetal force to the marble. As the ball rolled around the edge of the plate, the rim kept it moving in a circle. When the marble entered the cutout, there was no more force pushing it toward the center, and the marble traveled in a straight line across the tabletop. Something like this is probably what happens when the Earth goes around the sun. The Earth "wants" to keep moving in a straight line, but the force of gravity keeps it in a circular (elliptical) orbit.

SECONDARY EXPERIMENT

Materials

- A 12" ruler
- A strong rubber band
- A 2"-long small plastic tube
- Duct tape
- String, 15" long
- A bright piece of yarn, 2" long
- 2 or 3 heavy washers
- A watch with a second hand, and a friend to keep time

Preparation

1. Tape the tube onto the number side of the ruler so that one end of the tube is at the 0" mark and the other at the 2" mark.
2. Tie the washers firmly to one end of the string.
3. Pull the other end of the string through the tube, starting at the opening taped to the 0" mark.
4. Tie the string to the rubber band. Tie the yarn to the string/rubber band knot.

Procedure

1. Loop your fingers through the rubber band at the base of the ruler. Have your friend call out 8 second intervals
2. Start to swing the washers in a circle. Time it so that the washers pass the same point every 8 seconds.
3. Where is the colored yarn on the ruler? How many inches?
4. Have your friend call out 4 second intervals.
5. Time the revolutions so that the washers pass the same point every 6 seconds. Where is the colored yarn on the ruler now? How many inches?
6. Redo the experiment with more washers on the end of the string. What happens?

Results

When the washers were moving at one revolution every 8 seconds the colored yarn was at a lower number on the ruler than when it moved at one revolution every 6 seconds. When more weight (mass) was added, and using the same timing as the earlier experiment, the rubber band stretched a greater amount.

Conclusion

The faster the washers moved, the more the rubber band stretched. The faster the washers moved, the greater the centripetal force needed to hold it in orbit. As more mass was added, more centripetal force was needed to maintain the same number of revolutions per minute than with the lighter weight.

How a Foucault's Pendulum Works

Explanation

Ancient cultures believed that the Earth was the center of the universe and that all of the celestial bodies (the moon, the sun, the planets, and the stars) moved around the static (unmoving) Earth. They saw the sun rise above the horizon in the east, move across the sky to a position overhead at noon, and finally move to the opposite side of the sky, where it would sink to a point below the horizon in the west at nightfall. Since there was no feeling of movement, and the stars, sun, and moon were so small, people thought it was the sun and the stars that moved, not the Earth. Today we know that the Earth spins on its axis, much as a basketball spins while balanced on a basketball player's finger. It takes just about 24 hours for Earth to complete one full spin—called a revolution—on its axis.

Question

Before rockets and satellites went into space, how did scientists prove that the earth revolved on its axis?

Hypothesis

We can prove the earth moves on its axis with very simple tools.

Materials

- A strong cardboard carton, approximately 15" wide by 24" long by 12" deep
- A lazy-Susan turntable from a hardware or house wares store
- Cotton string
- A 3-ounce fishing weight
- Masking tape
- A ruler

Preparation

1. Place the turntable on a flat, stable service.
2. Have an adult help you cut off the 4 unsealed flaps of the carton.

3. Stand the box on one end (on the 15" x 12" side) on the middle of the turntable.
4. Tie a knot in one end of the string.
5. Securely tape the knotted end of the string to the top of the box at the open side.
6. Tie the weight to the end of the string. The weight should hang freely, 3" to 4" above the bottom of the box.
7. Test the pendulum action of the weighted string to make sure that the box doesn't wobble.
8. Place the ruler on the table directly in front of the weight and tape the ruler in place. The ruler will be used as a guide to measure the pendulum's path of swing.

Procedure

1. Hold the weight at its bottom with your fingers. There should be no slack in the string. Move the weight 8" forward, directly over the ruler. When the weight is released it should swing directly over the ruler.
2. Release the weight. When you are confident that the weight is swinging back and forth directly over the ruler, slowly turn the box/turntable approximately 10 degrees. Do not move the ruler. Is the pendulum still swinging in the same direction as when it first started?
3. Once again, slowly turn the box/turntable until it points approximately 45 degrees from the starting position. In which direction does the pendulum swing?

Results

The direction of the pendulum's swing should not have changed. It should still be swinging directly over the ruler.

Conclusion

A freely swinging pendulum always moves in a back and forth motion over its original path, despite any changes in the support's orientation.

In 1851, French scientist Jean Foucault (foo—KOH) proved that the Earth rotated by constructing a pendulum similar to yours. The two big differences between the one you made and the original is that his pendulum was 67 meters long (almost 220 ft.) and the weight at the end was 28 kilograms (almost 62 lbs).

Because the Earth is huge, we don't feel it rotating on its axis or traveling in its orbit around the sun—not to mention the whole galaxy spinning. When you look at a large "Foucault Pendulum," it appears that the pendulum's swing has changed direction. Actually, it is the direction of the surface of the Earth, including the land, buildings, trees, mountains, and oceans that have changed. Everything but the pendulum has moved.

NOTE: Have you ever sat on a train sitting in a station, right next to another parked train? Sometimes, if you look out of the window at the train alongside of you, it seems as though your train has started moving. Have you ever felt surprised to see the end of the other train pass you by, only to find your train is still sitting in the station? The same thing happens with a large pendulum arcing over the Earth or a smaller pendulum arcing over a turntable.

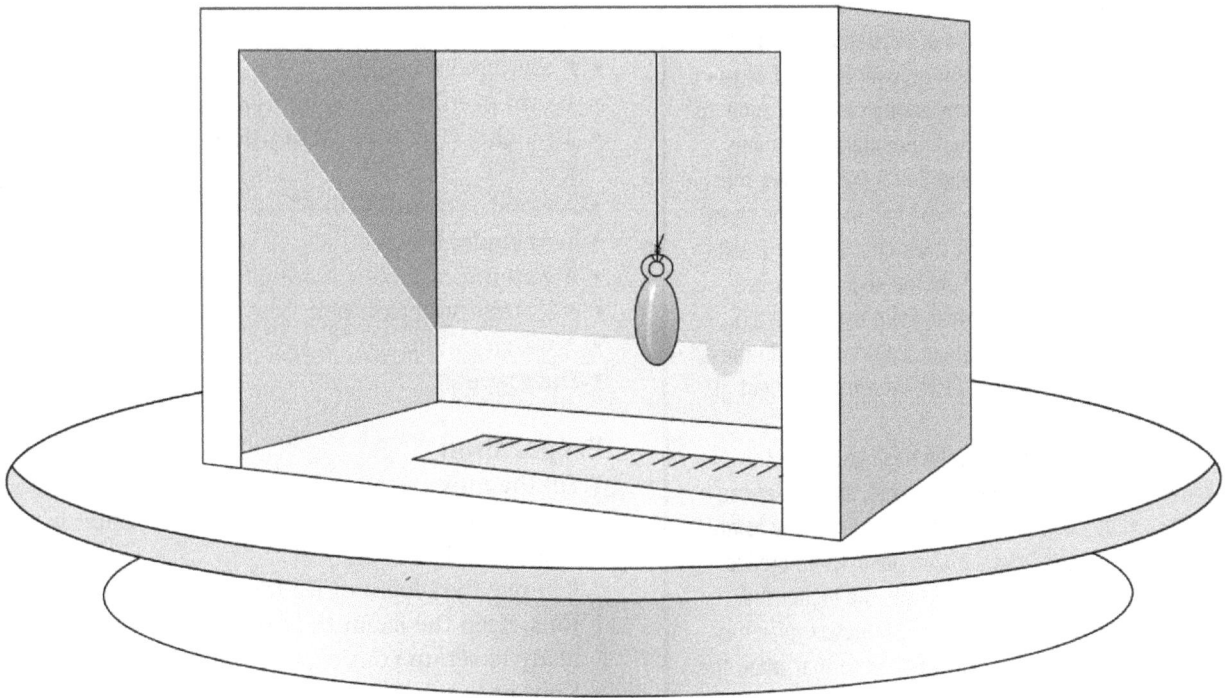

Skating on Thin Ice

Explanation
The three forms of matter are solid, liquid, and gas. There are many substances that can change back and forth quite easily. The most common is

---

BACKGROUND INFORMATION
When we walk on ice, we take very small steps to avoid falling down. If we try to slide on ice, we can skim along for two to three feet. Ice skaters seem to glide forever. How do they move so fluidly? Ice skaters glide over the ice because of a process called regelation (re-juh-LAY-shon). The skater's blade puts enough pressure on the surface of the ice to instantly melt the ice directly under the blade into a thin layer of water. This water layer allows the blade to slide as if on a frictionless surface. As the blade moves forward, the thin layer of water, no longer under the blade, refreezes instantly.

Let's look at this process of regelation and how it relates to glaciers. Glaciers form over a period of years when the temperature is low enough to allow snow to accumulate, generally in high mountainous regions and at the Earth's North and South Poles. There must be a sufficient quantity of snow fall, so that the snow does not melt or sublimate (turn directly from a solid to a gas) during precipitation. The snow banks get deeper and deeper every year, from tens of meters thick in small glaciers to about 1,500 meters in the largest glaciers in Alaska. More information about glaciers may be found at:

http://oceans-www.jpl.nasa.gov/polar/

When the proper conditions exist, the glacier can start to slide down hill, in much the same way as an ice skater glides across a frozen pond. The more ice and snow piled on top of a glacier, the higher the pressure underneath. Ice that is 50 meters thick has enough pressure at the bottom layer so that when the ice at the top layer is -7.6 degrees Farenheit (-22° C) or warmer, regelation occurs. The ice at the bottom layer turns to water and the ice above may start to slide downhill. As soon as enough ice moves away from the liquefied layer, the liquid turns back into a solid again.

---

water. When the pressure on water is about 14.7 pounds per cubic inch, (normal pressure at sea level) water takes the following forms: at 32 degrees Fahrenheit (0° C) and below, pure water is ice, a solid. Between 32 degrees and 212 degrees Fahrenheit (100° C), it is a liquid. Above 100 degrees Celsius, liquid water turns into water vapor—a gas.

Question
Does ice melt under increased pressure?

Hypothesis
Ice will melt when the pressure upon it is increased, and then will refreeze when the pressure is lessened.

Materials
- 2 clean, identical quart milk cartons
- Water
- A Styrofoam cooler
- 1 yard of thin (22 gauge) nylon monofilament
- 4 weights (1 pound each)—dumb bells are perfect
- A wooden board 3" to 6" wide by 2' long
- Two cinder blocks
- A waterproof table covering
- A leather or cotton belt
- A watch or clock
- Duct tape

Preparation
1. Fill the milk cartons with water. Place them in a freezer for about 48 hours, until the water is frozen solid.
2. Remove the blocks of ice from the milk cartons. Keep the ice in the freezer until you are ready to set up your experiment.
3. Knot one end of the monofilament around the handle of one dumbbell and tie the other end of the monofilament around the second dumbbell. There should be about 12" of monofilament between the dumbbells.
5. Tie the belt around the handles of the remaining dumbbells, one dumbbell at either end of

the belt. If you cannot tie knots tight enough to hold the dumbbells, use the duct tape. There should be about 12″ of belt between the dumbbells.

6. Spread the waterproof table covering on the tabletop.
7. Stand the cinder blocks on the table about 18″ apart.
8. Place the board across the cinder blocks. The board should be 10″ to 12″ above the tabletop.
9. Put the blocks of ice into the Styrofoam cooler.

Procedure

NOTE: Do this experiment in a cool area.

1. Remove the blocks of ice from the cooler and place them on the board.
2. Place the monofilament across one block of ice. The two dumbbells should be hanging down, one on each side of the board.
3. Place the flat belt across the other block of ice. The two dumbbells should be hanging down, one on each side of the board.
4. Note the time that you start.
5. Examine the blocks of ice and other equip-

ment, keeping notes on what is happening every five minutes.

Results

In a short time, the monofilament will be embedded within its block of ice. There is no open channel above or below the wire. There should be little to no change in the other block of ice. Eventually the monofilament will pass through its block of ice and rest on the wooden board. There is no evidence of an open cut in the ice block. There should be little or no evidence of penetration from the belt in the other block of ice.

Conclusion

The ice directly under the monofilament is under a great deal of pressure per square inch. Even though the same amount of weight was used with the belt and the monofilament, the width of the belt caused less pressure (lbs/square inch) on the ice than the thinner monofilament.

Pressure is determined by the amount of area of monofilament in contact with the ice times the weight. To make this calculation easy, let's

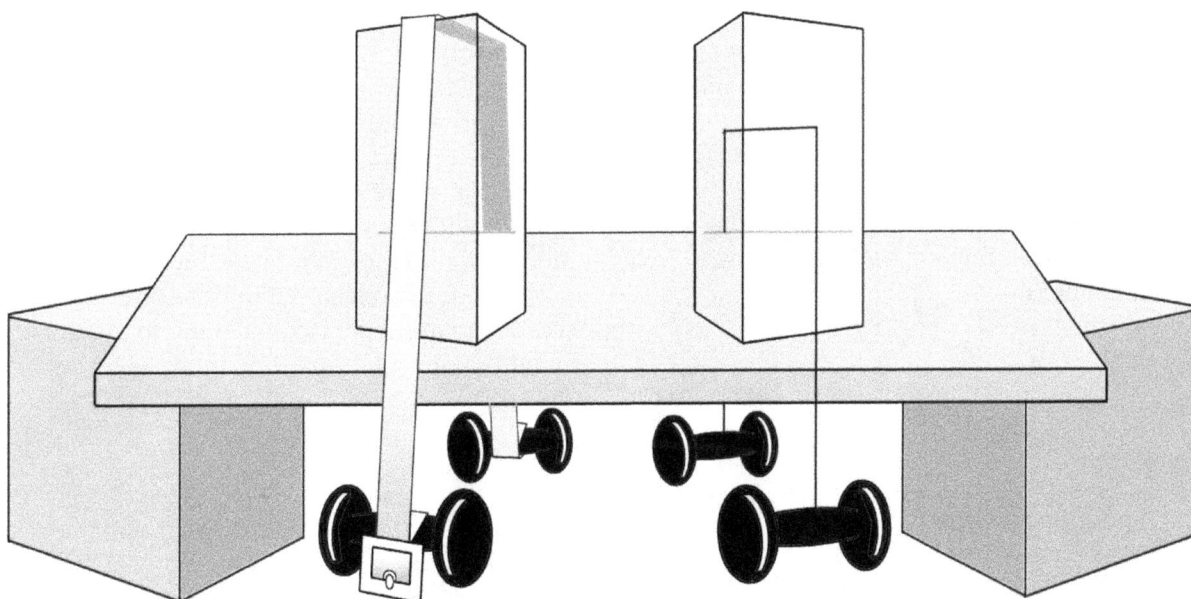

assume the wire is 1/50th on an inch in diameter. This means there is a maximum of 1/50th of an inch times the width of the block of ice at one time. If the ice is 10" wide, the total amount of wire touching it is only 10/50ths (⅕) of a square inch, or .20 in. The wire is weighed down by 2 lbs of dumbbell (we will not count the weight of the wire). That means that the pressure is about 10 pounds per square inch on the ice where the wire touches it. If the ice is only 5" wide, the pressure is 20 pounds per square inch. If it is less than 5" wide, the pressure is even higher.

If the belt is 1" wide, there is a total of 2 pounds of pressure on 10 square inches. Or .2 pounds per square inch. If the block of ice is only 5" wide, the pressure goes up to .4 pounds per square inch.

The much greater pressure under the wire causes regelation to occur. The monofilament melts the water directly beneath it. The wire goes through the liquid water and rests on the ice. The water on top of the wire re-freezes, and the ice under it melts. This happens continually until the wire has penetrated the block of ice.

SECONDARY EXPERIMENT

Use the same block of ice as above. You'll also need a small tin can of vegetables and a brick.

Procedure

1. Place the tin can upside down on the block of ice. The circular ridge surrounding the top of the can should be touching the ice.
2. Place the brick on top of the can.
3. When the rim of the can has sunk down into the ice, remove the weight and gently remove the can. Observe the results.
4. Replace the can and the brick on the ice.
5. After the can's rim has sunk into the ice, remove the brick, but allow the can to stay in place. Wait five minutes. Try to lift the can. What happens?

Results

The rim of the can sank into the ice until the top of the can touched the ice. When the can was removed, a circular impression filled with water could be seen. Within a few moments, the water turned back into ice. When the can remained without the brick, the can got stuck the ice.

Conclusion

The weight of the brick on the can caused an area of high pressure at the can's rim. When the flat top of the can touched the ice, the pressure (pounds per square inch) was lowered and regelation stopped. When the can was removed, the water refroze into ice. When the brick was removed and the can stayed in place, the decrease in pressure caused the water to freeze around the rim, and froze the can to the ice.

Playing with Perceptions

Explanation

There are many reasons why understanding the center of gravity is important. First, if we could not control our own center of gravity, we would always be falling down. In order to walk, run, skateboard, or ski, we need our center of gravity over our feet. A car with a low center of gravity is less likely to roll over. If an airplane's center of gravity were not considered during its design the plane would be unstable and hard to control. The same holds true for boats.

Center of gravity experiments and demonstrations can be non-intuitive. Some people call them discrepant (inconsistent) events. They just do not look possible. We will be experimenting with a few of these impossible looking happenings.

With your knowledge of the center of gravity, you can create events and experiments that defy the expectations and perceptions of people. You can record these experiments as qualitative studies: either a report on the affect the demonstrations have on people as observed by the experimenter or as a statistical report on how many people reacted one way or the other and why.

Question

Is it possible to control an object's center of gravity, so that it appears to move untouched by an outside force?

Hypothesis

It is possible to construct a device that has a changeable center of gravity that enables it to move, though untouched by a detectable outside force.

Materials

- A 3 minute egg timer (99 cent stores often have these)
- A small cardboard gift box, about 3" by 4" by 1" (Its diagonal measurement should be a bit longer than the egg timer.)
- Tissue paper
- Sticky tape

Preparation

1. Carefully remove the timer from its wooden cradle.
2. Place the timer into the box as in the illustration.
3. Pack tissue paper around the timer so that it can not rattle around.
4. Put the cover on the box.
5. Place a small pencil dot at both corners of the box where the ends of the timer are located.
6. Tape the box closed.
7. Stand the box on one edge, allowing the sand to run into the lower glass bulb.

Procedure

1. Position the box on its narrow side at a table's edge. Place the box so that ½ its width, the part with the timer's empty bulb, is just balanced as it overhangs the table's edge. Measure and record the length of the box's side hanging in space.
2. Wait for about 30 to 60 seconds. What happens? Why?
3. Do not allow any friends to open the box.
4. Ask them why they think the box fell from the table. Record their answers.
5. Try the experiment again but this time balance the box on the edge with the full sand-filled bulb at the bottom and record the length of the box's side hanging in space.
6. Compare the amount of lengths hanging in space in each case.

BACKGROUND INFORMATION

There was some talk years ago that Michael Jordan defied gravity with an excessive hang time when executing jump shots. He had a way of controlling his body, moving it around his center of gravity so that it seemed as though he was in the air for an unnaturally long time. Athletes who participate in the high jump and pole vault have a similar move, in which they twist their bodies around their center of gravity.

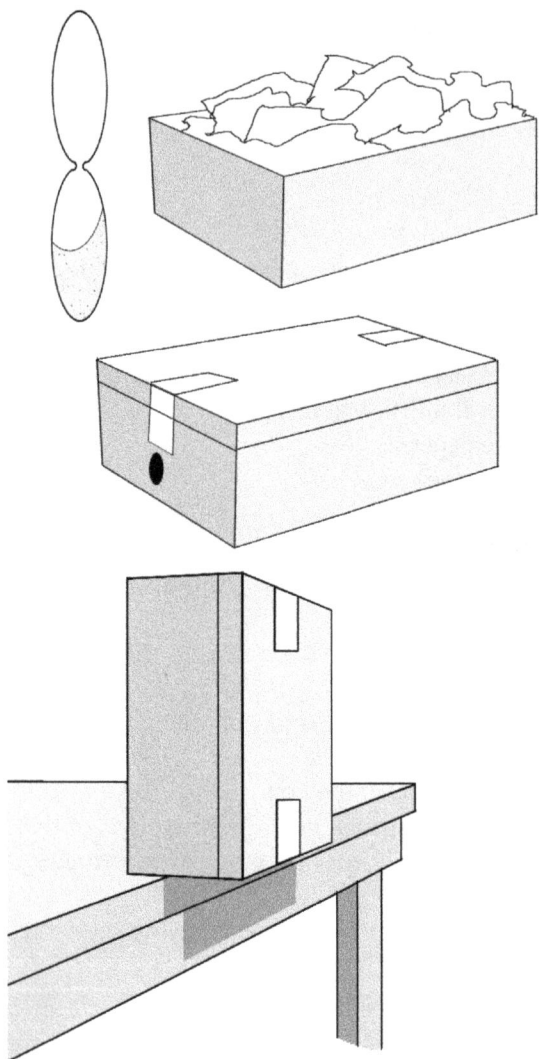

be more sand in the bottom bulb than the top bulb. At that point, the balance point of the box is hanging in mid-air over the edge of the table. The unseen force, gravity, pulls the box and everything in it to the floor. A shifting center of gravity does not generally spring to the minds of people as the cause making an object to fall.

SECONDARY EXPERIMENT

Question

Is it possible to make it appear as though an object is rolling under its own power, against the force of gravity?

Hypothesis

There is at least one method of manipulating an observer's perception and an object's balance point to make it seem as though an object is rolling uphill.

Materials

- 1 metal ruler
- A razor knife
- Sticky tape
- 1 heavy metal washer
- 4 identical cones (The cone's mouth should be at least 3" in diameter. The cones may be paper drinking cups that you sometimes find at water coolers or Styrofoam cones found in the crafts section of a department store. Tailors and dressmakers occasionally buy thread on large sturdy cardboard cones that would be perfect for this experiment.)
- 2 pieces heavy cardboard or foam core, 18" long

NOTE: Have an adult help you cut out the pieces for this project.

Procedure

1. Glue or sticky tape two cones together at their wide ends. Keep the cones aligned perfectly so that the rims of the cones don't overlap. This will be called the un-weighted cone. Repeat with the 2 remaining cones.

Results

The box should fall off table, when just balanced with the sand-filled bulb at the top. It should not fall at all when balanced with the sand-filled bulb at the bottom. If no one knows what is inside the box it is extremely difficult to figure out why the box fell.

Conclusion

When the sand is in the upper bulb, the center of gravity (balance point) of the box is on the table side of the table's edge. As the sand runs down from the top to the bottom bulb, the center of gravity starts to shift. Eventually there will

2. Tape the washer securely to the center line of one of the double cones. We will call this the weighted cone. The center line is where the cones meet.

3. Cut the heavy cardboard or foam core at 90 degree angles at both sides of the base. One short side will be 2" high, the opposite side 3" high. The top should be a cut as a straight line connecting the 1" and 2" sides. The straight line cuts should be as smooth as possible, with no gouges, dents, or mistakes to ruin the straight line.

4. Loosely tape the 2" ends of the cardboard together. The pieces should form a V. The 18" side will be on the tabletop. Separate the longer side with a small gap. We will call this the track.

Procedure

1. Place the center line of the un-weighted cone between both walls of the track at the lower end.

2. Slowly separate the higher ends of the track.

3. There will be a moment when something strange happens. What is it and why do you think that occurs? Does center of gravity have anything to do with this?

4. Keep on experimenting to find the optimal spacing that allows the event to occur.

5. Measure and record the height above the table of the double cone's pointed ends when it is at the short end of the track and at the high end of the track. What are the results? At which location are the pointed ends higher above the table top? At which point lower?

6. Measure and record the optimal distance to enable the experiment to work most easily. This will help you easily set the apparatus up at any time.

7. Set the optimal distance that the two 3" sides should be from each other.

8. Attempt the procedure with the weighted double cone, keeping the washer down toward the table. What happens?

9. Ask some subjects how they think it is possible for the double cone to be rolling uphill. Record their answers.

Results

When the shorter ends of the track are at the proper distance from each other, the washer-free cone will start to roll from the shorter side to the taller side. It is apparently rolling uphill. The weighted cones will not roll uphill.

Conclusion

Though it seems as if the un-weighted, double cone is rolling uphill, that is not the case. The center of gravity or balance point of the double done runs point to point. The pointed ends of the cones (center of gravity) are a greater distance above the table top when at the short end than at the higher end. Even though it seems as though the cones are rolling uphill, the center of gravity is moving downward as shown by the measurements.

The weighted cones do not roll because the taped-on washer has moved the center of gravity from between the pointed ends to a point near the rims where the cones meet. The center of gravity of the cones is already at a low point and cannot roll uphill against gravity, no matter how far we separate the track's ends.

Crime Scene Investigation

Explanation

Many police departments use a process called chromatography to identify substances found at a crime scene. Chromatography separates the chemicals in a mixture. It can prove or disprove that a particular chemical mixture such as ball point pen ink on a ransom note is or is not the same as the ink in a pen owned by a suspect. Chromatography is based on the fact that various molecules making up mixtures and compounds vary in size and weight. This sounds technical but this procedure is really quite easy to do right on your kitchen table. All you need is porous paper and a solvent and the samples to be tested.

Question

Can we actually separate substances into various colors that when combined give it a distinctive hue?

Hypothesis

Using paper chromatography, we can differenti-

ate between various inks from different pen manufacturers.

Materials

- A large, clean coffee filter
- Scissors
- Sticky tape
- Various black marking pens (Sanford, Sharpie, Flair, Staples store brand, magic Marker)
- A large glass measuring cup
- Various solvents (water, nail polish remover, rubbing alcohol)
- A ruler
- A pencil
- A stapler
- A watch
- Safety goggles
- Rubber lab gloves

SAFETY NOTES:
- **Wear goggles and gloves when doing this experiment.**
- **Make sure that there is adequate ventilation when using solvents.**
- **Do not use solvents in the presence of an open flame**

Preparation

1. Cut the filter paper into strips 6" by ½".
2. Using the ruler, draw a straight pencil line across each strip ½" from one end.
3. Make a ?" fold in the other end of each strip.
4. Place the folded end over the pencil. Staple the paper together, forming a tube, so that the pencil will not fall out.
5. Fill the measuring cup with enough solvent so that when the pencil is laid across the mouth of the measuring cup, the solvent will reach the pencil line and no higher. Try water first. If that does not work, try rubbing alcohol and then acetone (nail polish remover)
6. Label the top of each strip in pencil with the name of one brand of pen.
7. Make a mark/dot with each pen, about ⅛" above the pencil line on the strip identified with that pen's name.

BACKGROUND INFORMATION

Scientists who want to identify the component chemicals of growing leaves or leaves that have changed color in the fall use chromatography. You can even use this process to find out what kind of food coloring was used to make your favorite jellybeans.

A sample of the mixture under investigation is placed on the filter paper, near but not touching an edge. The edge of the paper is placed in the solvent. The solvent travels through the paper by capillary action. As the solvent travels, it dissolves the mixture. The chemicals that make up the sample material move through the paper with the solvent. Certain parts of the dissolved chemical will move more slowly than other chemicals in the sample and the pure solvent. This difference in speed causes the chemicals to separate on the paper. Specific chemical mixtures have color patterns that are constant and replicable, assuming the solvent, the paper, and the time are the same.

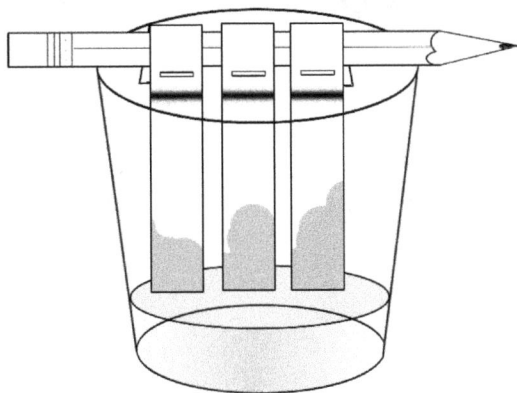

8. Place the pencil over the mouth of the measuring cup. The solvent should reach only as high as the drawn pencil line. Through capillary action, the solvent will move up the paper. Do not allow the ink dot to dip into the solvent.

9. Allow the solvent to touch the paper for exactly 30 minutes. The time measurement must be exact for each ink mark. We already know that the paper and the solvent are identical for each sample.

10. Remove the samples from the measuring cup and allow them to air dry.

Results

Each sample should have different chromatographs. Generally, the lengths and colors of the lines on the filter paper will all be different.

Conclusion

Each company uses a different formula to make black ink. We can tell that by the way the chromatograph is made up of colors in various patterns.

SECONDARY EXPERIMENT: Part One

Use the same materials as above.

Procedure

1. Have a friend make a mark on a piece of filter paper with one of the pens.

2. Proceed with the chromatography process using this unknown ink blot and the same solvent. Allow the process to go on for exactly 30 minutes.

3. Compare the mystery blot to your samples.

Results

One of the original samples should be an exact match for the mystery sample.

Conclusion

Chromatography is a process that allows us to compare substances and match identical substances with high accuracy.

SECONDARY EXPERIMENT: Part Two

You know that a friend came to your house, rang the doorbell, then ran away. You do not know who it was. The only evidence that you have is a smudge of green on the door. You do know that your three best friends eat different types of green candy. How can you find out which one of them was at your door?

Procedure

1. Lightly dampen the green smudge with water.

2. Rub a coffee filter strip on the smudge, about $1/2$" from the bottom of the strip.

3. Perform a chromatographic examination of the sample.

4. Get a sample of the candies that each of your friends eat.

5. Lightly dampen each piece of candy and rub it on a filter paper strip, $1/2$" from the bottom.

6. Perform a chromatographic examination on each piece of candy.

Results

One of the strips should match the mystery sample strip.

Conclusion

You will know who left the smudge on your door and you can say, *"Busted!"*

Exploring the Möebius Strip

Explanation

There is a part of mathematics that involves surfaces called topology. The people who study this area are interested in what happens when we move across, twist, or bend surfaces. This is a part of geometry and can be fun to study. There are many unexpected happenings that seem impossible.

We know that if we cut a piece of paper in half, we will have two pieces of paper. We also know that when we form a strip of paper into a loop and cut right down the center line of the strip, we will have two loops, or will we?

Question

What will happen if I create loops of paper, some with twists, and some without, and cut them down the center line?

Hypothesis

It is possible to construct loops of paper so that when they are cut along the centerline, unexpected results will happen.

Materials

- A roll of white adding machine tape, 3" wide
- Sticky tape
- Scissors

Preparation

1. Cut three 34" strips from the roll of adding machine tape.

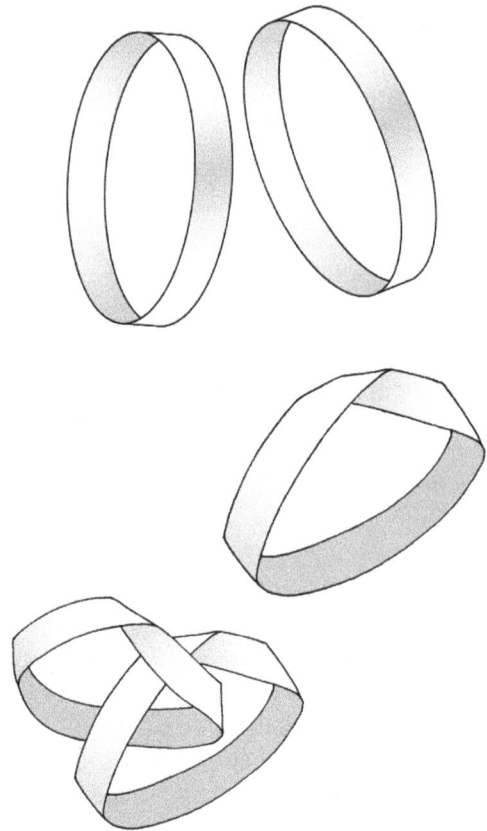

BACKGROUND INFORMATION

The father of topology is thought to be a Swiss mathematician named Leonhard Euler (pronounced LE-nard OI-ler). Another important explorer of mathematical surfaces is a man by the name of August Ferdinand Möebius (MOW-bee-us) who was not content to examine flat surfaces but studied the results of putting twists in surfaces. He came up with some spectacular results.

---

2. Turn one of these long strips into a loop by taping the two free ends together.
3. Lay the next strip stay flat on the table. Twist one end so that the top side becomes the bottom.
4. Use the tape to join the ends. This will give you a loop with a half twist in it. This is called a Möebius strip.
5. Leave the final strip flat on the table. Twist one end so that the top side of one end is now the bottom side, just like before, but now give it a second twist, in the same direction.
6. Tape the ends together to make a loop with a full twist.
7. If you wish, make a number of additional sets of all these loops so you can repeat the experiment.

Procedure

Use the same procedure when cutting down the center line of the three loops.

1. Pick up the loop and use the scissors to cut it down the center, so that each remaining strip will be 1" wide.
2. Track and record the way the loop was constructed, your hypothesis, and the actual results.
3. How many strips do you think you will have?
4. Will they be regular or will they have a twist in them or be odd in some other way?

Results

Loop One (no twists): two normal loops

Loop Two (half twist): one long loop with a full twist

Loop Three (full twist): two loops of equal size, but they are twisted and looped through each other

Conclusion

When an untwisted loop is cut through its center line, the result is two separate loops. When a loop with one twist is cut through its center line, the result is always one long loop twice the length of the original. When a loop with one full twist is cut through its center line, the result is two interlocked loops.

SECONDARY EXPERIMENT

As you have seen, Möebius strips are extremely odd, which makes them lots of fun. When we think of something like a piece of paper we "know" that it has two surfaces, top and bottom, or front and back. It doesn't seem possible, but Möebius strips are objects with only one surface, though we think we see and feel two. Try this next experiment.

Materials

- 3 strips of white paper, 3" by 34"
- A pencil or crayon
- Scissors
- Sticky tape
- A ruler

Preparation

Place the three strips of paper on the table and make three loops (no twists, a half twist, and a full twist) as in the first experiment.

Procedure

Draw a line with the crayon along the center line of the untwisted loop until the crayon line meets itself at the beginning. Draw a line along the center lines of the half twisted and full twisted loops. Ask the following questions:

1. What do you think will happen?
2. If the strip is 34" long, how long will your crayon line be?
3. What happens when you reach the 34" mark, just by the starting point?
4. How long is the entire drawn line?

Results

The plain loop with no twist should have a line that is 34" long on one side of the paper. The loop with the full twist will have a 34" line that follows the paper strip's twisted surface.

The Möebius Strip is the interesting one. When you draw the 34" line along the center line of the strip, your crayon is on the opposite (what you might call the bottom) side of the paper. As you continue to draw the line, it will move back to the original (what you might call the top) side of the paper and connect with the line's starting point.

Conclusion

Möebius strips exhibit strange qualities. Though it seems as though there are two surfaces, top and bottom, there is really only one. This is difficult to grasp because you can feel the top and bottom. Yet by drawing a line down the center line, you've proved that not only is there a single surface, but it is twice as long as you would suspect upon casual observation.

Möebius strips have a practical application. They are used as conveyer belts that move items from one place to another. Since the working surface of the belt is twice as long as a similar belt without a twist, the surface takes longer to wear out. The Möebius belt can be serviced or replaced less often than an untwisted belt.

Junkyards, Doorbells, and Pinball Machines

Explanation: The magnets that most of us see every day are the buttons that hold your drawings and family photos to the refrigerator door. These are permanent magnets. There is another kind of magnet that is in junk yards, automobiles, pin ball machines, and even in most houses: electromagnets.

An electric current flowing through a wire wrapped around a piece of iron, such as a nail or a screwdriver blade, turns the iron into an electromagnet. Electric currents and magnetic fields interact with each other in ways that we frequently find useful. Not only does an electric current cause a magnetic field, but also a copper wire passing through a magnetic field causes an electric current to happen.

Electric currents are said to have a positive (+) and negative (-) side. Take a look at an unplugged lamp, toaster, or hairdryer. The plug has at least two blades, one positive and the other negative. If there is a third prong, usually a circular rod, we say the cord or appliance is "grounded," meaning it is highly unlikely that someone will get a shock if the appliance is used as recommended. Magnets do not have positive and negative sides, but they do have north and south poles. North and south is different from positive and negative, but there is a connection.

Question: Can an electric current actually turn something into a magnet?

Hypothesis: An insulated copper wire carrying an electric current, when wrapped around a piece of iron, can turn the iron into a magnet.

Materials
- A large dry cell lantern battery (You can find at Radio Shack or a camping store)
- An insulated spool of 18-gauge copper wire, 10' to 20' long
- A small single-pole double-throw switch that visibly shows "ON/OFF" (Radio Shack)
- A wire stripping tool
- A wire cutting tool
- A wooden handled screwdriver with a 6"-long blade
- A 10" piece of copper pipe or tubing
- A 10" piece of aluminum tubing
- A box of iron paperclips
- A penny
- 2 ten-penny carpenter's nails
- A pair of pliers
- An 8 ounce can of soda.
- String
- Masking tape
- A small camera tripod or microphone stand

Preparation
1. Remove the wire from the spool. Do not allow it to get tangled.
2. Using the wire cutting tool, cut one piece, about 1' long from the wire's end.
3. Use the wire stripping tool to remove 1" of insulation from the four ends of the wires.
4. Attach one end of the short wire to the switch. Make sure the switch is in the "OFF" position.
5. Attach the free-end of the short wire to one terminal on the battery.

Procedure
1. Wrap five turns of wire around the center of the screwdriver's blade. Wrap from the middle of the long piece of wire.
2. Attach the free end of the long wire to the unused battery terminal.
3. Put the paperclips and the penny on the table.

BACKGROUND INFORMATION

Junkyards use electro-magnets for picking up massive pieces of iron, such as wrecked cars. Automobile starter motors have an electro-magnet in the piece called the solenoid. Pin ball machines have many of them. The flipper button has an electro-magnet that allows you to keep the ball in play. All the gimmicks that push the ball out of holes and the hammers that kick the ball away from the mushroom-like posts use electro-magnets. When someone pushes the button at the front door of your home, electric doorbells generally have an electro-magnet that activates the chime or buzzer.

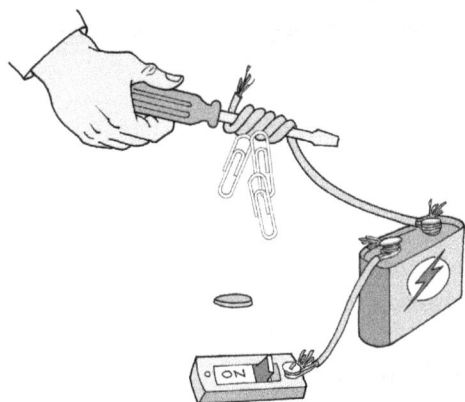

4. Move the switch to the "ON" position. Holding the screwdriver's handle put the blade tip on top of a penny. Raise the tip above the tabletop. What happens?
5. Move the tip of the blade to the paperclips and raise the tip above the tabletop. What happens?
6. How many paper clips, using only the blade's end, did you raise at one time?
7. Move the switch to the "OFF" position.
8. Wrap another ten turns of wire around the center of the blade. Move the switch to the "ON" position and touch the paperclips. How many paper clips, using only the blade's end, did you raise at one time?
9. Wrap the wire around the center of the aluminum tube and repeat the above experiment. What happens?
10. Wrap the wire around the center of the copper tube and repeat the above experiment. What happens?

Results: The aluminum and copper tubes wrapped with wire did not pick up any paper clips. The screwdriver wrapped with wire did not pick up the penny. The screwdriver wrapped with wire did pick up some iron paper clips. The more turns of wire around the blade, the larger the number of paper clips that were picked up.

Conclusion: When current flows through an insulated copper wire which is wrapped around an iron screwdriver blade, the blade can act like a magnet. The greater the number of turns of wire, the stronger the magnetic pull. When the switch was turned off, the screwdriver ceased to act like

a magnet. The magnet picked up iron, but not the copper or zinc penny. Current carrying wire wrapped around aluminum or copper tubing does not cause the tubes to become magnetic.

SECONDARY EXPERIMENT

NOTE: Must be done with adult supervison

Preparation: Do not do this step of the experiment yourself. Ask an adult to hold the nails in an open flame until they become red hot, and then allow them to cool slowly. This is an annealing process, which will remove any residual magnetism in the nails. When the nails are cool to the touch, you can make the following preparations.

1. Tie the head of each one to a piece of string.
2. Tie the strings together so the nails are hanging at the same height.
3. Form a coil of wire by wrapping the long length of wire around the soda can. Keep the ends of the wire free.
4. Slide the coil from the can. Hold the coil together using two small pieces of masking tape wrapped around opposite sides of the coil.
5. Attach the coil to the switch and battery, with the switch in the "OFF" position.
6. Assemble the tripod. Hang the nails from the center of the tripod, so they are centered within the coil, but not touching the table top.

Procedure
1. Move the switch to the "ON" position. What happens?
2. Move the switch to the "OFF" position. What happens?

Results: When the current is flowing, the nails separate and touch opposite sides of the coil.

Conclusion: This is similar to what happened in the first experiment. The current flowing through the coil magnetized the nails. The nails were magnetized in the same way, the north and south poles assuming the same position on each nail. Similar poles repel each other, so the nails flew apart.

Good and Bad Vibrations

Explanation

Resonance occurs when the vibrations of one object moves at the identical natural frequency of another object, making that other object vibrate. Some people explain resonance as the reinforcement of vibrations. When you play a musical instrument, such as a piano, violin, or guitar, resonance occurs on the other keys, the soundboard, or within the resonating cavity, giving the sound a louder, richer sound.

Resonance in musical instruments is a good thing. In the case of The Tacoma Narrows Bridge in Washington State it was not. A number of factors, including resonance, caused this bridge to collapse.

Opened in 1940, this suspension bridge quickly received the nickname Galloping Gertie. Whenever the wind blew at a sufficient speed, the bridge's roadway would start to gyrate and buckle. People would drive or walk across the bridge while it was dancing wildly, as though it were an amusement park ride. One day the wind was blowing at 35 miles per hour. For three hours, the resonant vibrations of the roadway had 1½ feet of amplitude (height). When the wind increased to 42 miles an hour, the cables and roadway could no longer take the strain. Galloping Gertie's main span collapsed and crashed into the waters below.

Similar things have happened when soldiers march across a bridge. Occasionally, if they are all in step, a bridge will start to resonate, and the roadway will buckle and wave. Because of that, marching soldiers usually break cadence when crossing a bridge.

Question

Can resonance be observed under laboratory conditions?

Hypothesis

Resonance, the reinforcement of vibrations, can be observed in the laboratory using simple equipment.

Materials

- A 5' tall camera tripod
- String
- A weak magnet
- A large, clean, empty tin can
- A one pound weight that can fit in the can
- A yardstick

Preparation

NOTE: Have an adult help you with these preparations

1. Use a can opener to remove the top of the can.
2. Ask the adult to drill or punch 4 equidistant holes around the can's opening.
3. Tie a separate 5' length of string through each hole.
4. Open the tripod to its full height.
5. Tie the strings to the center of the tripod. The can should be hanging from the tripod, close to, but not touching the floor. You have constructed a pendulum.
6. Put the weight in the can.
7. Place the yardstick under the center of the tripod.
8. Tie a separate 5' piece of string to the magnet.

Procedure

1. Put the magnet on the can.
2. Pull the string quickly. What happens?
3. Put the magnet back on the can.
4. Pull the string gently in the same direction as the yardstick, and then allow the string to go slack. (Do not pull hard enough to disengage the magnet.)
5. Allow the can to swing back and forth.
6. As the can swings back toward you, pull the string gently enough so that it does not disengage from the can. Once again, allow the string to go slack. What happens? (This should add a bit of energy to the pendulum and the swing should swing back and forth in an arc, a tiny bit larger than before.)
7. Continue this gentle pull and release of the

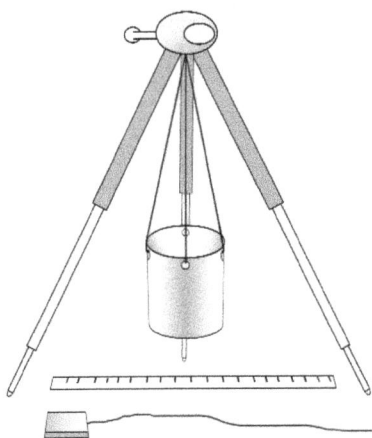

string for three minutes. How long has the distance traveled by the pendulum in one to-and-fro motion become?

8. Repeat the experiment, but after the can is swinging, pull the string as the can is moving away from you. What happens?

9. **Extra Credit Question:** When you have stopped adding energy to the system by pulling on the string, does the frequency (the time that it takes for one full back and forth motion) change as the length of the arc changes?

Results

The length of the tin can's arc should have increased bit by bit when you pulled on the string as the can came toward you. When the string was pulled as the tin can moved away from you, the magnet detached itself from the can.

Extra Credit Answer: The frequency will be the same no matter what the length of the pendulum's swing.

Conclusion

We can add energy to a system (the tin can pendulum) a bit at a time, as long as the system's natural frequency is met. When the frequency is different, (pulling the string as the can moved away) there is no increase in the system's energy.

SECONDARY EXPERIMENT

Energy can be added to a system with a push as well as a pull.

Use the same set up as above, but instead of pulling with a magnet, push the pendulum with an outflow hose from the exhaust of a canister vacuum cleaner. Place the hose into the outflow port of the vacuum cleaner. Position the vacuum cleaner so that the hose can easily reach the pendulum.

Procedure

1. Start the vacuum cleaner.
2. Put your hand over the end of the hose so that little air escapes.
3. Place the covered hose's end near to, but not touching the pendulum.
4. Allow the air stream to hit the can for one minute. How far away from dead center does the can move?
5. Allow the can to stop swaying.
6. Put your hand over the end of the hose so that little air escapes.
7. Place the covered hose's end near to, but not touching the pendulum.
8. Remove and replace your hand from the end of the hose.
9. As the can swings away, allow the air stream to hit the can.
   When the can reaches the top of its swing away from you, cover the end of the hose.
10. Continue this procedure for three minutes, always covering the hose as the can reaches the top of its "away" swing. What is the result? How far did it move at first? How far was it moving at the end?

Results

The can moved away from you a little bit when you pointed the hose at it for one minute. When you aimed the air stream at the can as it moved away, stopping the stream as it came toward you, the distance the pendulum moved continued to increase.

Conclusion

Resonant vibrations can be set up in a system by the force of the wind (air streams). Resonance, along with other factors, was the cause of the collapse of the Tacoma Narrows Bridge.

Free Fall and Weight

Explanation

Free fall happens when an object is falling or moving under the influence of no force other than gravity. Down here on the ground, we have a force pushing us up that equals the force of gravity. If there were no force pushing us up, we would fall through the Earth. The force of the Earth pushing us up is called the normal force.

When a skydiver jumps out of a plane, she is in free fall, until the force of the air pushing up stops her from accelerating. Sometimes we can feel the effect of free fall in an amusement park. When you are on a large roller coaster, the first drop—the one that makes you feel as though your stomach has been left behind—is very close to free fall. If you could rig up a scale to weigh yourself on that roller coaster, your apparent weight would be much less than it would be on solid ground.

BACKGROUND INFORMATION

Sir Isaac Newton, famed British Scientist having nothing to do with the cookie bearing his name, came up with a useful explanation of gravity in 1643. Gravity, as defined by Newton, is an attractive force (each object attracts another) between two objects. Earth attracts the moon, and the moon attracts the Earth. The Earth attracts us, and we attract the Earth, only the Earth is so much larger it seems as though we are at the mercy of the gravity of Earth.

In 1905, Einstein changed the concept of gravity. His theory of relativity explained that gravity was actually a warping of space. Imagine a rubber sheet with a bowling ball in the middle. A smaller ball is spinning around the bowling ball at a velocity that keeps it from falling into the middle, yet not fast enough to move out of the heavy ball's depression. (Please note that the rubber sheet concept is just an analogy and is a way for us to visualize the concept. Space is not a rubber sheet.)

Question

What happens to us in free fall?

Hypothesis

Weight is meaningless in free fall.

Materials

- A paper coffee cup, 4" high
- 2 rubber bands, 3" long
- 2 rubber bands, 3" long but lighter weight than the above
- A paper clip
- Sticky tape
- 6 large metal washers
- 2 2-ounce lead fishing weights
- A sharp pencil

Preparation

1. Punch a hole in the center of the cup's bottom.
2. Push the 2 heavier rubber bands partly through the hole in the cup's bottom.
3. On the outside of the cup, hook the paper clip through the rubber bands so they cannot slip back through the hole.
4. Tape the paper clip flat to the bottom of the cup.
5. Attach 3 washers to each of the rubber bands. Push the bands through the holes in the washers and secure them as in the illustration. The washers should be on the inside of the cup.

Procedure

1. Pull each set of washers from the cup and allow them to hang over the cup's lip. The sets should be on opposite sides of the cup.
   NOTE: The washers should be heavy enough to keep the rubber bands from pulling them into the cup.
2. Stand on a small step ladder (be careful).
3. Hold the cup in front of you.
4. Drop the cup and observe what happens to the washers.

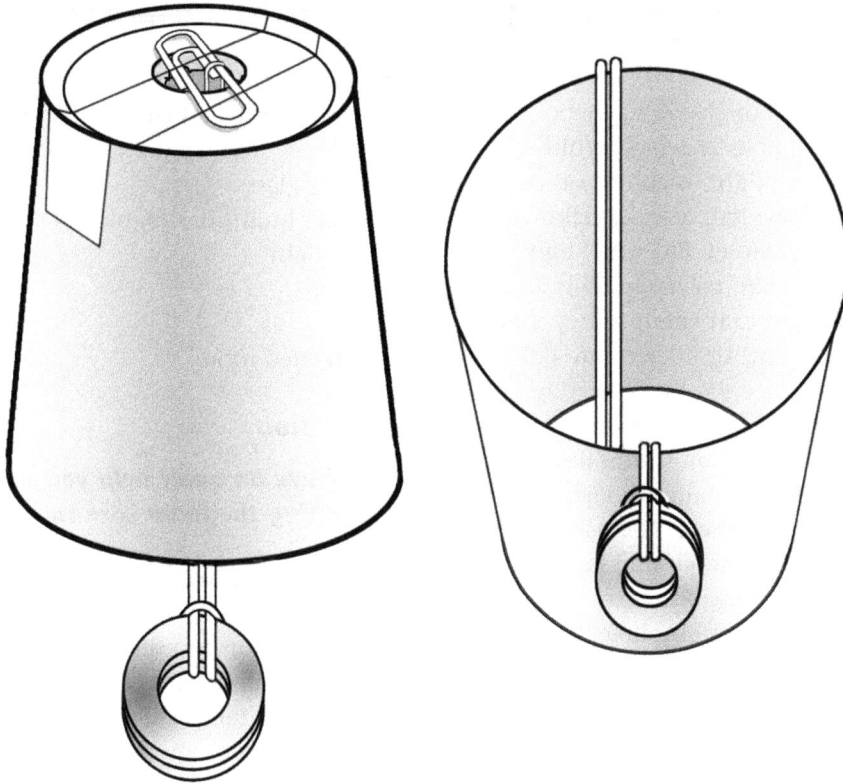

5. Record what happens.
6. Change the weights to heavy fishing weights and repeat the experiment using the heavier weights. Record the results.
7. Change the rubber bands. Use the thinner rubber bands of the same length. Repeat the experiment using the weaker rubber bands and record the results.

Results

You should observe the washers drawn into the cup regardless of the weights used and the strength of the rubber bands.

Conclusion

Gravity, with an assist from friction at the cup's lip, pulls the weights down, with a force stronger than the force of the rubber bands pulling the weights into the cup.

When the cup is dropped, the entire construction is in free fall. The cup, rubber bands, and the washers/weights are all falling and accelerating at the same rate. Gravity is acting equally on all of the pieces. In free fall, the force of the rubber bands pulling on the weights does not have to fight against gravity, so the weights are pulled into the cup. In free fall, the washers and fishing sinkers are basically weightless. But remember: they still have the same mass as before you dropped the cup. The weight changes, but the mass does not.

Properties of Light

Explanation

Visible light is composed of electromagnetic waves that our eyes are able to detect. White light, which includes sunlight, is composed of all the colors of the rainbow: red, orange, yellow, green, blue, indigo, and violet. But white light hits our eyes less often than colors do. This is because most of the light that enters our eyes has been either refracted (bent) or filtered into colors.

Light moves in straight lines unless it is reflected or refracted. As the sun shines down on us, the light waves, after traveling through empty space, hit the atmosphere. There are extremely small particles of solids and liquids suspended in the atmosphere. The scattering of sunlight going through the atmosphere, the blue rays in particular, is so great that on a clear day the sky looks blue.

Question

Why are sunsets red?

Hypothesis

When white light passes through a filtering medium, such as the atmosphere at sunset, the blue waves are scattered more than the red, allowing more red rays for us to see.

BACKGROUND INFORMATION

The sky is frequently red at sunset. The Earth is a globe (ball) surrounded by a 600-mile bubble of gas called the atmosphere. As the Earth revolves on its axis and the sun appears to sink in the West, the sun's rays have to travel through the atmosphere at an extreme angle. This means they are traveling through much more air—40 times more than when the sun is overhead—and hitting many more particles. The atmosphere acts like a lens and bends the sunlight. Not only are red rays refracted less than blue and green rays, many of the blue and green rays are scattered and filtered by the particles in the air. So, our sunsets are red.

Materials

- A tube made of a foam core and black masking tape
- A water glass
- A small, bright flashlight that shines with a white light
- Water
- Milk
- A darkened room

Preparation

NOTE: Have an adult help you when constructing the foam core tube.

1. Cut 4 strips of foam core, approximately 12" by 24".
2. Tape the strips into the shape of a hollow tube. Cover the edges with the black masking tape to make the tube as light proof as possible.
3. Cut a foam core square, 14" by 14".
4. Put three or four drops of milk in the glass and fill it with water.
5. Place the tube on its side on a sturdy, flat surface.
6. Place the glass inside the tube, near one end.
7. Turn on the flashlight and shine it through the glass into the tube. Look inside. Notice the color of the milky water.
8. Cover the end of the tube where the glass sits with the square piece of foam core, blocking out light from the room.

    Hold the flashlight and shine it into the open end of the tube so that it illuminates the glass. What color is the liquid now?

Results

The water should have a reddish tinge when the flashlight is shining through the glass and a bluish tinge when the light is hitting the front of the glass, which is darkened behind.

Conclusion

When the light shines through the glass, the particles of milk suspended in the water scatter and absorb some of the blue light. When that hap-

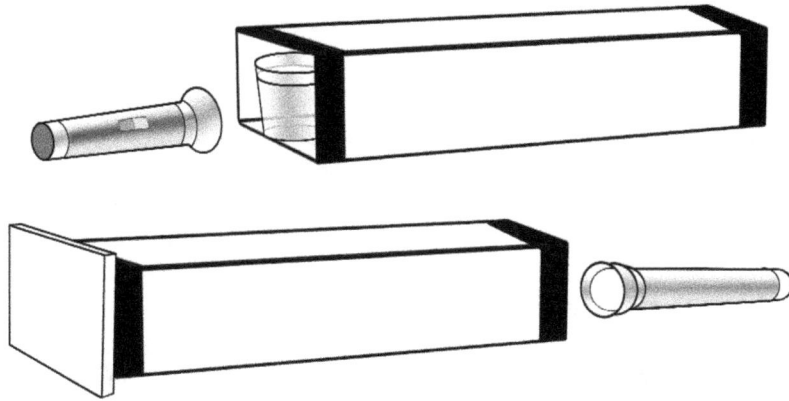

pens, the milk appears to have a red tinge to it. This is probably what happens when sunlight goes through the atmosphere at sunset, and sunsets appear red.

When the light shines on the front of the glass, the particles scatter more blue rays than red. As those blue rays of light scatter and some are reflected back into our eyes, they travel a shorter distance than when the flashlight was behind the glass. When the sun is shining between sunrise and sunset, the blue rays get scattered much more than the red rays, giving us blue skies.

SECONDARY EXPERIMENT

Unless an object creates its own light (such as a light bulb, candle's flame, or the sun) we only detect objects by sight when light reflects from them. If the object absorbs all of the colors, it will appear black. Frequently objects will absorb various colors of the spectrum and only reflect one or more colors. When we see a red car in sunlight, the car's paint has absorbed all the colors but red. The light reflected from the car enters our eyes and we see a red car. When we see green grass, all the colors except green have been absorbed. A white object, like a brand new baseball, the inside of a cream filled cookie, or a wedding dress, reflects all the colors.

Question
How do pigments determine the color of an object?

Hypothesis
Pigments absorb light waves of all of the colors in white light, except for the actual colors of the pigment, which the pigment reflects.

Materials
- At least 7 different bright colored crayons in the colors of the rainbow: red, orange, yellow, green, blue, indigo, and violet.
- The tube from the Light Waves experiment
- A small, bright flashlight that shines with a white light
- Lighting gels, or filters—if you can only get one, make it either red or green. Purchase gels from local theatrical lighting companies or maybe from your school's theater department. If all else fails they can be found at www.scientificsonline.com
- A piece of heavy black felt 36" by 36"

Preparation
1. Cover one end of the tube with the square of foam core, holding it in place with a bit of tape. The more light, the better.
2. Cut the gels into pieces that will totally cover the lens of the flashlight, letting no white light escape.

Procedure: Part One
1. Place the crayons into the open end of the box so the colors are readily visible.
2. Hold the flashlight in one hand.
3. Place your face near the opening of the box. Cover your head with the piece of felt. No

light should be leaking into the tube or under the felt. What do you see?

4. Turn the flashlight on and shine it on the crayons. What do you see?

Results

When there was no light allowed into the box, the inside of the box was black, and the crayons could not be seen.

When the flashlight was switched on, the crayons could be seen, and each color could be identified. The felt was still black, and the inside of the tube was black or at least a very dark shade of gray.

Conclusion

When light is absent, nothing can be seen. Black objects are black in the dark and when light is present. When light is shone on objects, the objects will absorb all of the colors except for the color of the object which is reflected. That is why we see a red crayon as red and a green one as green.

Procedure: Part Two

1. Fit the red gel over the flashlight. It might need to be held in place with the tape. Don't forget! There should be no white light visible when you switch the flashlight to the "on" position.

2. Duck under the felt one more time with the flashlight off.

3. Turn on the flashlight and shine it on the crayons. What do you observe?

4. Replace the red filter with the green filter. What do you observe?

Results

When the red filter is on, the red crayon is visible, and the green crayon appears black. When the green filter is on, the green crayon is visible, and the red crayon appears black.

Conclusions

When a red light illuminates a red object, and there is no other light source, the object is visible. When the same red light falls on a green object, very little light is reflected, and the object appears to be black. When a green light illuminates a green object, and there is no other light source, the object is visible. When the same green light falls on a red object very little light is reflected, and the object appears to be black.

Some objects (in this case crayons) have pigments (the colors that reflect light) that are made up of more than one color. These are partially visible in filtered light.

How to Measure a Charge

Explanation

What do a bolt of lightning, a shock from walking across the carpet, clothes sticking together in the dryer, and a balloon sticking to the wall have to do with each other? They are all examples of static electricity. The study of these and related phenomena is called electrostatics.

Inside an atom of normal matter, protons (positively charged particles) and electrons (negatively charged particles) are relatively close together. The positive and negative are equally matched, and the charges generally cancel each other out. (Like charges repel each other and unlike charges attract each other.)

Pulling or separating these positive and negative charges within an object (ionization), results in what we call static electricity. One way to charge items is by rubbing them with the appropriate fabric. Not all combinations of materials and object can create a charge. In everyday usage, some materials will rarely retain a charge. Static charges when noticeable, generally involve voltages of between 1,000 and 50,000 volts. However, this voltage is involved with little to no current (amperage). When you rub a balloon on your hair to get it to stick to a wall, you create a charge of well over 10,000 volts. These everyday charges are generally harmless to humans because there is no amperage involved.

WARNING: Never experiment or play with high amperage electrical current without expert supervision

BACKGROUND INFORMATION

When Benjamin Franklin flew a kite in a thunderstorm, he was very lucky. Many books tell us that he discovered that lightning was electricity when lightning hit his kite. His experiment involved detecting a charge from the air on the kite's string. If lightning had struck the kite or string, he probably would have died a painful, unattractive death.

Question

How can we prove that like (2 positive/2 negative) charges repel each other and unlike (positive/negative) charges attract?

Hypothesis

If similar charges repel each other, we can test for that by attempting to place two similarly charged items near each other and observing the results.

Materials
- A cork
- A sewing needle
- Scissors
- A piece of wool fabric (such as an old wool stocking cap, a wool sock, or a wool muffler)
- A plastic soda straw

Preparation
1. Cut the straw in half.
2. Pierce the exact center of one of the short straws with the needle. The hole should go through only one wall of the straw. The straw should be able to spin on the needle.
3. Remove the needle from the straw.
4. Stand the cork on one end.
5. Push the eye of the needle into the cork's top.

Procedure
1. Hold the wool fabric firmly around the straw.
2. Build up a charge on one end of the straw by pulling the straw through the fabric 5 times.
3. After the fifth stroke, do not let go of the straw. You should be holding the straw's end with the wool fabric.
4. Pick up the cork and needle with your other hand.
5. Still grasping the straw with the fabric, place the needle in the pre-made hole.
6. Stand the cork on end so the straw can swing around in an unrestrained manner.
7. Note which end of the straw has been charged (rubbed with the wool).

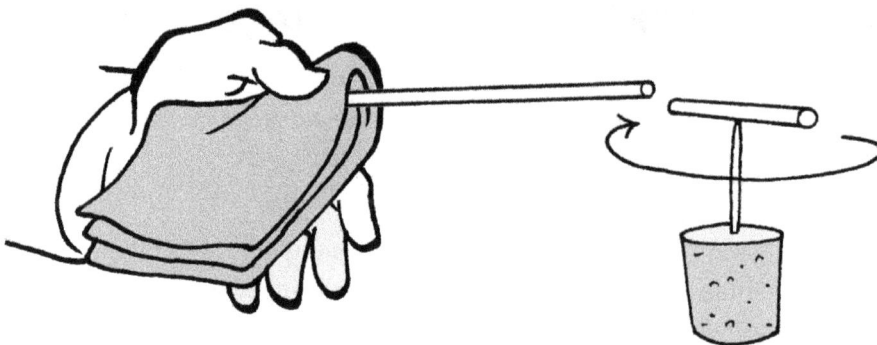

8. Build up a charge on one end of the second straw with the wool fabric.
9. Do not allow the straws to touch each other.
10. Bring the charged end of the straw in your hand near the uncharged end of the straw on the needle. What happens?
11. Bring the charged end of the handheld straw near the charged end of the straw on the needle. What happens?
12. Rub your fingertips up and own the handheld straw.
13. Bring the straw near both ends of the straw on the needle. What happens?

Results

When the charged straw approached the uncharged end of the straw on the needle, there should be no obvious effect.

When the charged straw approached the charged end, the straw on the needle should swing to the side, away from the straw in your hand.

When you rubbed your fingers on the straw (causing the straw to discharge) and brought it near the needled straw, there was no obvious effect.

Conclusions

When similarly charged (plus or minus) articles approach each other, the similar charges repel each other.

When a charged item approaches an uncharged item, there is no apparent repulsion.

When a charged item is discharged (the positive and negative portions are no longer separat-

ed), there is no apparent repulsion by either charged or uncharged items.

SECONDARY EXPERIMENT

Is it possible to detect electric charges without getting zapped? We can detect electric charges, both positive and negative, with a simple instrument.

Materials

• Thin aluminum foil. Regular household foil is probably too heavy to work well. Thin foil from a stick of chewing gum's wrapper will work best. Carefully peel the foil from the

---

BACKGROUND INFORMATION

Charges, both positive and negative, can be detected by using an electroscope. Jean Antoine Nollet invented the electroscope in 1748. Two years later Abraham Bennet invented the gold-leaf electroscope. Since then, various metals such as aluminum have been used to make leaf electroscopes. Electroscopes have two leaves (extremely thin pieces of a conducting metal). In the presence of a charge, the two leaves have a similar reaction and they separate. Upon removing the charge, the leaves move back together. The original electroscopes used gold foil. Gold is malleable, which means it can be easily shaped by pounding it with a hammer. Gold can be beaten into sheets 1/250,000 of an inch thick. To put it another way, some gold foil is so thin that if held up to a light, you can see through it.

paper. An easy way to do this is to soak the foil in some hot tap water that has a few drops of liquid dish soap mixed in. After a brief period of time, maybe 15 minutes, place the foil, paper side up on a flat plate. Gently rub the paper side of the wrapper. The paper should detach itself from the foil a little bit at a time.

- A metal paper clip
- A clear plastic soda cup
- Scissors
- A pair of needle nosed pliers
- A variety of plastic, glass, and rubber substances (soda straws, ball point pens, combs, rubber and mylar balloons, a pencil, a plastic sandwich bag)
- A variety of fabrics (cotton, wool, polyester, poly/wool, linen, silk, paper)

Preparation

1. Ask an adult to help you pierce the bottom of the cup, making a hole the same size as clip's diameter. Your adult assistant may use a small drill bit, an awl, or the tip of a hot melt glue gun.
2. Cut the foil into strips. Each strip should be about ?" by 1 ?."
3. Open the paper clip so that it resembles a J.
4. Align the two pieces of foil and pierce one end of the combined strips. Keep the shiny sides of the foil facing each other. (If there is a residue of adhesive on the paper side, it might keep them from moving freely.)
5. Slip the foil onto the J end of the clip.
6. Turn the cup mouth-side down.
7. Insert the tail end of the J through the hole in the cup's bottom, from the inside of the cup. Push the clip up until the ends of the foil are above the cup's mouth.
8. Bend the part of the paper clip extending from the cup at a right angle so it will not fall through the hole.
9. Put another right angled bend in the clip so the end stands upright.
10. The J arm of the clip and the foil should not touch the cup's walls.

Procedure

1. Note and record the object and fabrics used in each part of the experiment.
2. Pick up the straw. Touch it all over with your fingers. Touch the straw to the end of the paper clip
3. Pick up the soda straw and rub it five times with wool.
4. Bring the straw near to, but not touching, the paperclip's end. What happens?
5. If the foil leaves separate, put the straw down and touch the end of the paperclip with your fingers. What happens?
6. Continue testing each piece of fabric with the straw. Keep a record of which fabrics charge the straw and which do not.
7. Test each object, one at a time, with each fabric.

Results

When brought near the point of the electroscope, certain items, when rubbed with certain fabrics, caused the leaves to separate.

- This did not happen with every combination of item and fabric.
- You will have a list of which fabric can charge each item.
- Silk rubbed on glass gives an opposite charge to wool rubbed on a soda straw.

Conclusion

The rubbing together of certain items, such as a soda straw and wool, separated the positive and negative electric charges within the straw. As the straw neared the electroscope, the straw induced a charge (gave a charge to the clip without losing its own charge) in the paper clip and the foil leaves. Because both leaves had the same charge, they were forced apart. When a finger touched the point of the electroscope, the positive and negative charges were evenly distributed throughout the foil. Gravity pulled the leaves downward, where they hung side by side.

Make Your Own Rainbow

Explanation

There is a folktale about a pot of gold at the end of the rainbow. We know that this is only a story because when we approach a rainbow, it moves. It's impossible to reach out and touch it.

British scientist Sir Isaac Newton made many discoveries. One of these was about light. He figured out that although bright sunlight appears as white or perhaps yellow, it actually consists of all of the colors of the rainbow and then some.

Newton curtained off a window, leaving only a small hole. When sunlight came through the hole, Newton positioned a table and a prism (a solid crystal with equal-shaped sides) so that the sunbeam would enter one face of the prism, bend, or refract, and when leaving a different face of the prism, shine on a white background. He discovered that sunlight could be broken down into seven observable colors.

He went one step farther and blocked off all the colored light from the prism but blue. He passed the blue light through another prism expecting to see it broken down into more colors. He found that the blue portion of sunlight was composed of only one color. He discovered the same for all of the other colors too. The seven basic colors were primary—they could not be broken down anymore.

Question

Will a prism separate white light into the colors of the spectrum?

Hypothesis

White light can be separated into the seven primary colors of the spectrum with a prism.

Materials

- A glass or plastic equilateral prism (all the sides and angles are the same) You can find one at: www.scientificsonline.com
- A bright light source such as a white flashlight or high intensity lamp
- 2 pieces of cereal box cardboard 4" by 10"
- Black masking tape
- White cardboard 12" by 8"
- 2 lumps of clay
- Crayons
- Talcum powder

Preparation

1. Score the white cardboard 4" up, parallel to the 8" edge. When bent at the score, the cardboard should be able to stand upright. This will be your viewing screen.
2. Place a lump of clay about 4" from the cardboard.
3. Balance the prism on one edge of the clay. The edges of the prism should be parallel to the white cardboard.
4. Place the second lump of clay 4" to 6" from the prism.
5. Bend the two pieces of cereal box cardboard in half, forming two 5" high tents.
6. Place the tents between the lump of clay and the prism.

NOTE: Depending upon the brightness of your light source and the quality of the prism, these distances may be increased.

Procedure

1. Turn off all of the lights in the room.
2. Turn on the flashlight.
3. Place the flashlight on the clay pointing toward the white screen. Adjust the flashlight's position so that the light enters the prism.
4. Adjust the two cardboard tents between the flashlight and prism so that a portion of light shines between them. The tents will block the rest of the light.
5. Use the black masking tape to create a horizontal slit between the two tents. If done properly, there will only be a horizontal sliver of light hitting the prism.
6. Adjust the position of the prism by rocking it back and forth on the edge that is in the clay. You want the light hitting the screen to break up into many colors.
7. Observe and record the colors of light shining

on the screen. Write down the order of the colors as you see them, from top to bottom. Which color is on top? Which is on the bottom?

8. Draw a picture or take a photo of the apparatus.

9. Blow a very small amount of dust (talcum) from your palm into the space between the prism and the screen. You should be able to see the paths of each light color. Which color bends the most? The least? Why do you think the spectrum is wider than the line of light entering the prism?

10. On a separate piece of paper, draw a side view of the apparatus, including the paths of the various colored lights as they go from the prism to the screen. Use the crayons to indicate the various beams.

Results

White light entered the prism as a thin horizontal bar. When it left the prism, the beam was wider and broken up into many colors. The talcum powder made the various colors visible.

Conclusion

White light is composed of light beams of at least seven visible colors. When a beam of white light goes through a prism, it breaks up into its constituent colors. The visible colors are red, orange, yellow, green, blue, indigo, and violet.

The red portion of the white light bends the least and the blue portion the most. Due to the varying amounts of bending for each color in the spectrum, the light on the screen is wider then the horizontal bar entering the prism. The orientation of the prism determines if red is on top or bottom.

SECONDARY EXPERIMENT

In addition to the materials from the preceding experiment, you will need a second prism. Place prism #2 with the flat face down and an edge facing up. The first prism faces in the opposite position. Hold any face of prism #2 directly next to the face of prism #1 where the light exits. What do you see? What happens to the spectrum? Hold prism #2 a short distance (?″) from prism #1. What happens to the spectrum on the screen?

Results

In both instances, the spectrum was replaced with a white light.

Conclusion

White light consists of light waves of many colors. Different colors of light are bent different amounts when they enter and then leave a prism. These colors can be both separated from white light and reassembled into white light by prisms.

Electric Circuits

Exploration

We turn on electric appliances, including lights, every day. But how does the switch send an electric current to the light bulb, television, or toaster? Electric currents flow along wires, or circuits, uninterrupted by gaps. This is useful because we can summon electricity simply by turning on a switch. The switch, when flicked on, assures a continuous circuit. When flicked off, it puts a gap in the circuit. Electric wire (generally copper) is filled with electrons (subatomic particles) from one end to the other. When we hook up a source of electricity (a wall socket or battery) to one end of the wire, put an instrument (a light bulb, refrigerator, or computer) on the other end, and a return wire to the source of electricity, electrons flow from the source through the wire to the instrument and back to the source. This happens so quickly that it seems to be instantaneous. If we use a switch somewhere in the middle, we don't have to be constantly connecting and disconnecting wires for the electricity to flow.

BACKGROUND INFORMATION

There are two categories of electricity. First, there is static electricity, which we feel as a shock when we cross a carpet and touch a door knob. Static means "not moving." This type of electricity can produce lightning, but it does not generally produce a flowing current. The second category is composed of electric currents that flow. That flow of current can be from a battery, a generator, a magnet, a wall socket, or even a photocell, which is powered by sunlight and then powers televisions, computers, and toys. Electric currents are AC (alternating current) or DC (direct current). AC is supplied to our houses by public utilities (electric companies). The most common supply of DC is found in dry cell batteries such as D cells, AA cells, or AAA cells. Direct current is also produced by the wet-cell (lead-acid) batteries found in cars and trucks.

Question

Can a simple series circuit work if there is a gap in the wiring?

Hypothesis

A simple series circuit must be unbroken in order to work properly.

NOTE: This experiment must be performed with adult supervision. Do not touch any electrical circuits, plugs, or wires in your home!

Materials

- A block of balsa wood (2" by 4" by 1")
- Unpainted silver metal thumbtacks (not push pins)
- Sandpaper
- A metal paper clip
- A small spool of 18 or 20 gauge insulated copper wire (Radio Shack)
- 4 small light bulbs, the kind that screw into a flashlight (Radio Shack)
- 4 sockets for the light bulb (Radio Shack)
- 2 battery holders, each to hold 2 AA cells (Radio Shack)
- 4 AA cells
- A needle nosed pliers with a wire cutter jaw
- A wire stripper or pliers with a wire stripping groove
- 2 flat pieces of plywood, 15" by 15"
- Double sided foam tape (hardware store)

Preparation

Make two switches as follows:

1. Scour the top of three thumbtacks with the sandpaper.
2. Cut two 1 foot lengths of wire from the spool. Use the wire stripper to remove about 1" of insulation from the ends of both wires.
3. Use the needle nosed pliers to wrap one end of each wire around the points of each thumbtack.
4. Use the needle nose to grab the inner loop of the paper clip and pull it outside of the larger loop.

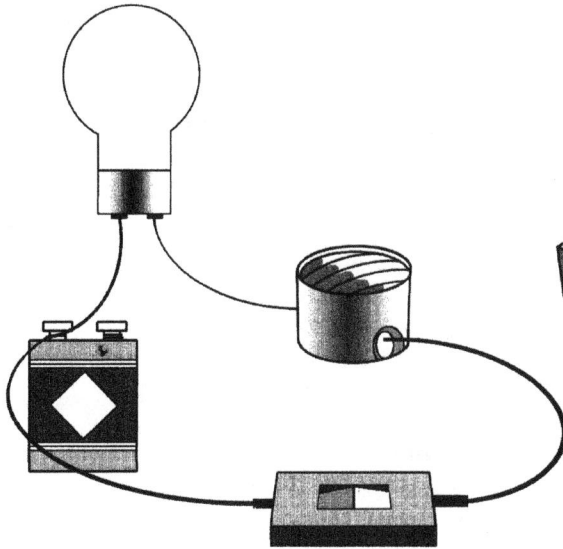

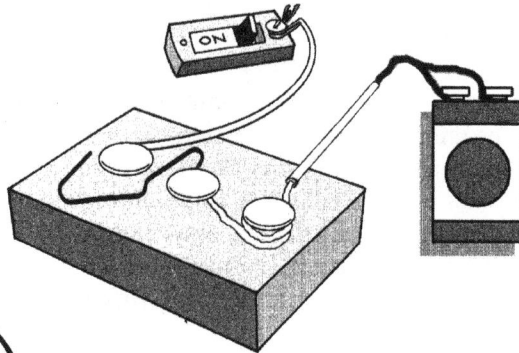

5. Push one tack with its wire into the block.
6. Push the other tack with wire through one end of the paper clip and then into the block.
7. The second tack should be positioned so that the paper clip's free end, when pushed down, touches the top of the first paper clip. The clip's springiness will allow the end to move up and break contact with the tack when you stop pressing with your finger. You have just constructed the first electrical switch.
8. Next, place the following components on the flat piece of plywood in the positions shown in the illustration. Attach the 4 items (not the wires) to the plywood with the double sided tape: 1 battery holder, 1 switch, 2 lamp sockets, 4 pieces of wire.
9. Have an adult help you strip lengths of wire and attach them in this order:
   - A wire goes from one end of the battery pack to the switch.
   - A short wire runs from the switch and connects at one side of a bulb holder.
   - A second short wire connects both sockets.
   - A final piece of wire goes from the second bulb holder to the free end of the battery pack.
   - Install the batteries.

Procedure

1. Press the switch down, completing the circuit. Do both bulbs light up?
2. Unscrew either bulb. Press the switch. Does the remaining bulb light up?
3. Reverse the bulbs, screwing the loose one in and loosening the one that just worked. Does the remaining bulb light up?
4. Screw in both bulbs and try the switch. Do the bulbs light up?

Results

With both bulbs in place and the switch pushed down to complete the circuit, both bulbs should light up. When one of the bulbs is removed from its socket and the switch is pushed down, the remaining bulb does not light up.

Conclusion

For electricity to flow in a series circuit, a complete, unbroken connection must be maintained. When there is a gap in the circuit, for any reason (the switch is open, one bulb is unscrewed or burnt out) the remaining lights will not glow. In order for electrons to flow from one end of a wire to the other, a complete circuit is necessary. This is the reason that some Christmas tree light sets stop working until the burnt out bulb is replaced.

SECONDARY EXPERIMENT

The series circuit is useful, but limited. If that were the only way to build a circuit, and one light bulb burned out in your house, all of the other bulbs in the house, the TV, the refrigerator, and all other appliances would stop working too. A parallel circuit enables all the other components to work, even if one of them is broken or missing.

Question

Can we make a circuit that will work if one bulb is burned out or missing?

Hypothesis

A circuit can be constructed that will allow all the other bulbs to work, even if one of them is removed or burned out.

Preparation

Use the same components as you did for the first experiment. Lay the battery holder, switch, 2 lamp sockets, and 4 pieces of wire on the plywood. Attach with the double sided tape.

1. Hook up two 4" pieces of wire to each bulb holder.
2. Connect one end of the switch to the battery holder with a 6" piece of wire.
3. Attach a 6" piece of wire to the free end of the battery pack.
4. Attach a 6" piece of wire to the other end of the switch.
5. Connect one socket to the ends of the wire from the battery pack and the switch.
6. Prepare two more 6" pieces of wire by stripping both ends of both wires.
7. Hook a wire to each side of the remaining bulb holder. Attach the free ends of the wires to the connection marked "X."
8. Install the batteries and bulbs.
9. Press the switch to test the circuit. If both bulbs light up, the circuit is complete.

Procedure

1. Unscrew either bulb.
2. Press the switch. What happens?
3. Screw in the loose bulb and unscrew the other one. Press the switch. What happens?

Results

No matter which bulb was unscrewed the remaining bulb lit up when the switch was depressed.

Conclusion

A parallel circuit is a little more difficult to make than a series circuit, but when one bulb burns out, the other bulb stays lit. The electrons will flow in the unbroken portion of the circuit. This must be how the wiring in our homes and schools is designed, since one burnt-out or switched-off appliance usually does not affect the others.